Lower Urinary Tract Dysfunction - From Evidence to Clinical Practice

Edited by Ran Pang

Published in London, United Kingdom

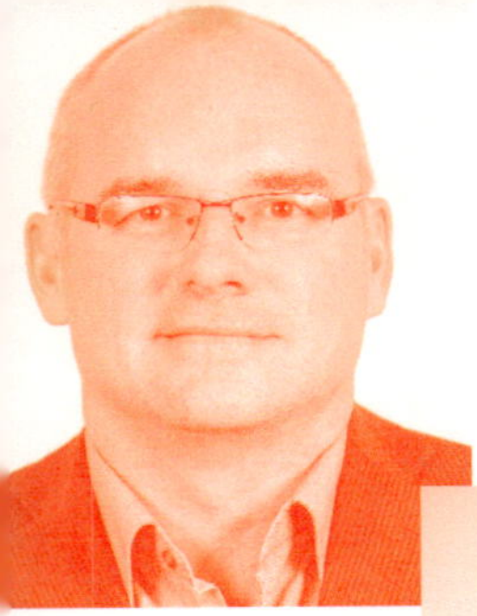
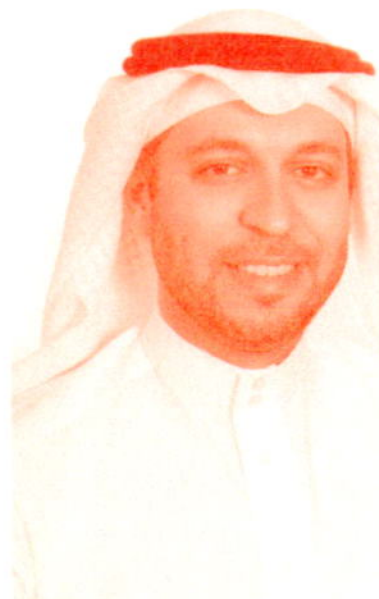
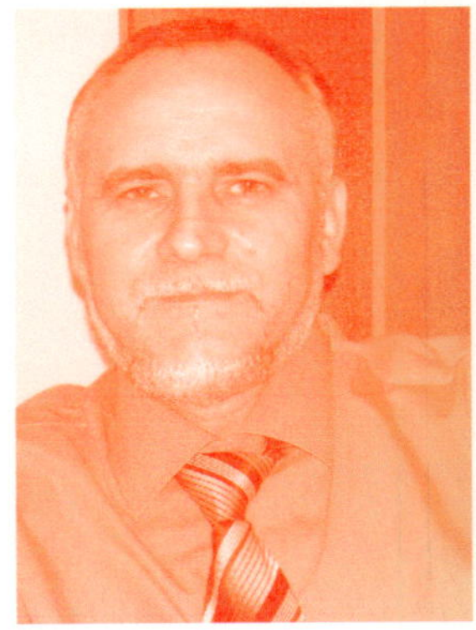
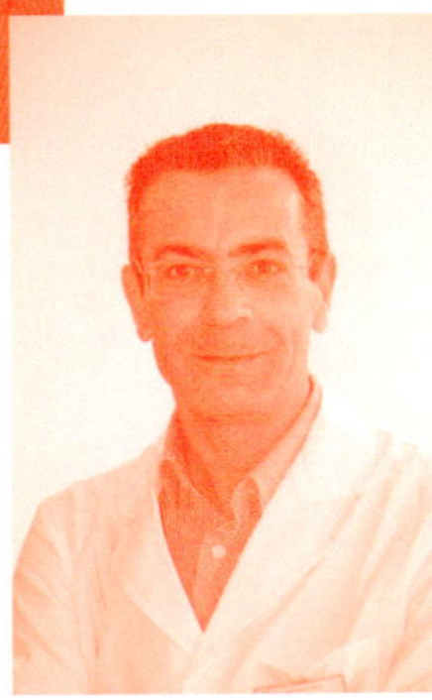
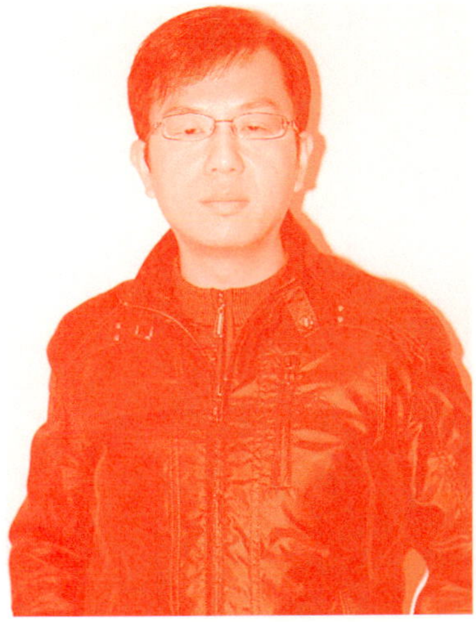
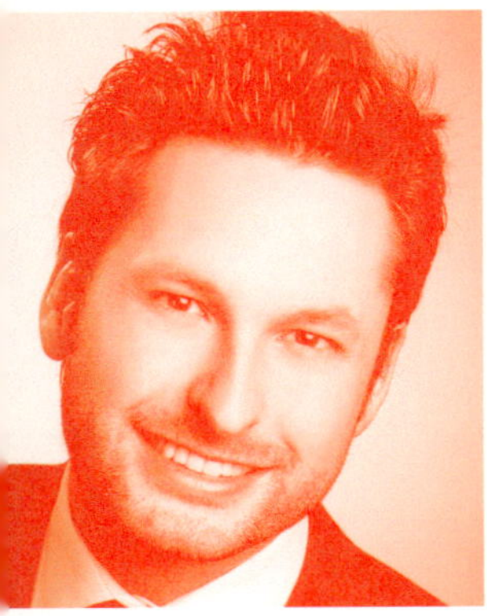
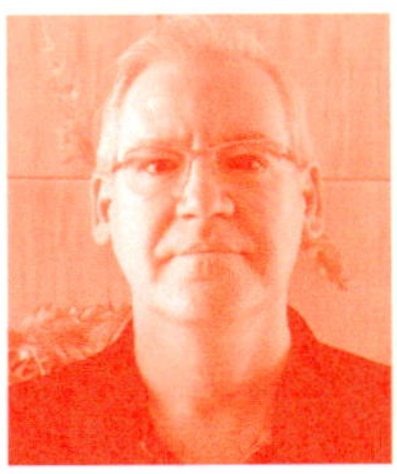

IntechOpen

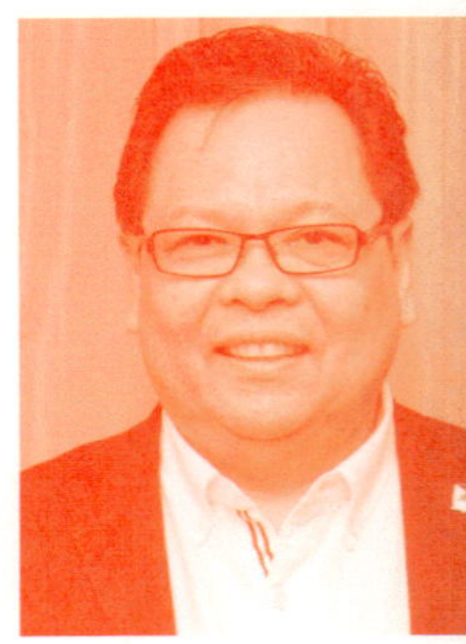
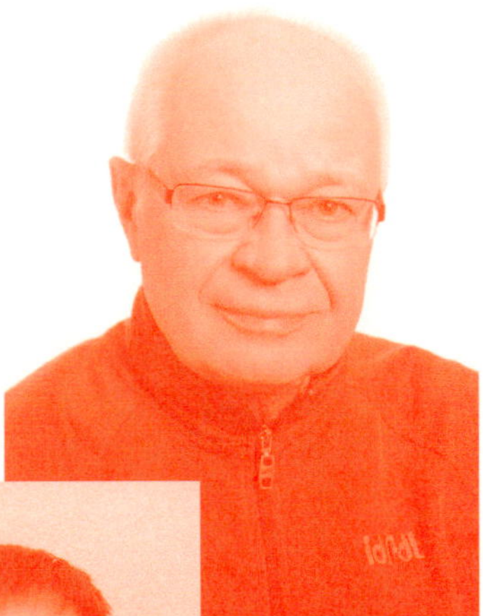
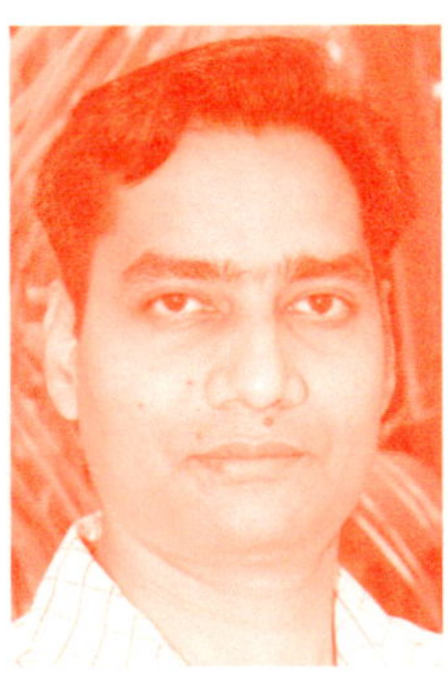
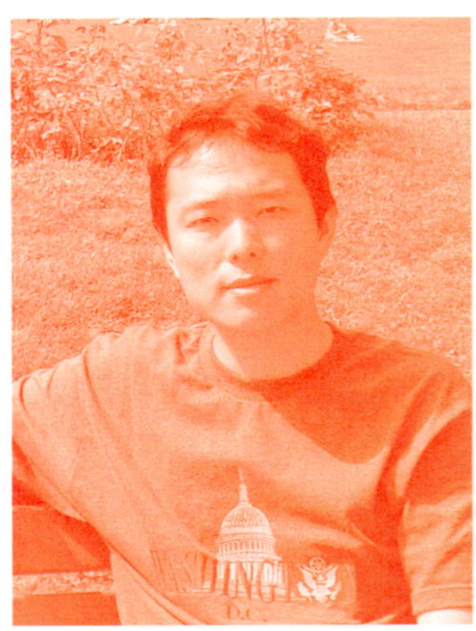
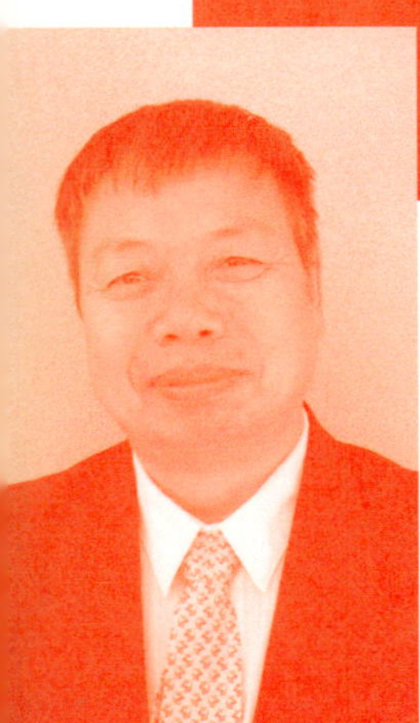
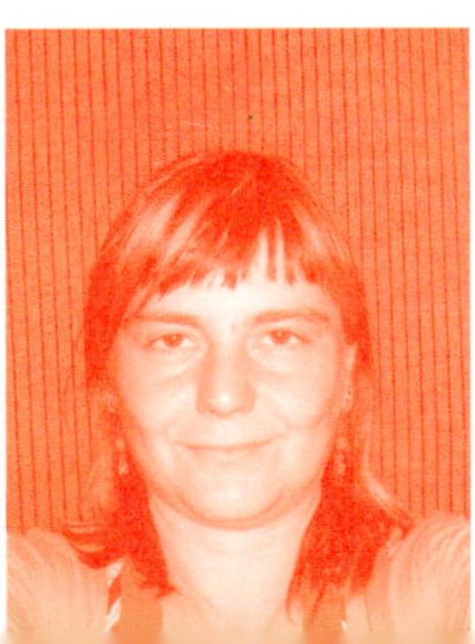

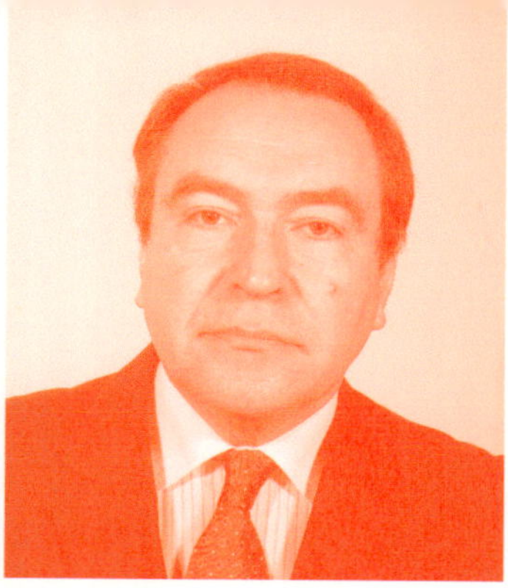
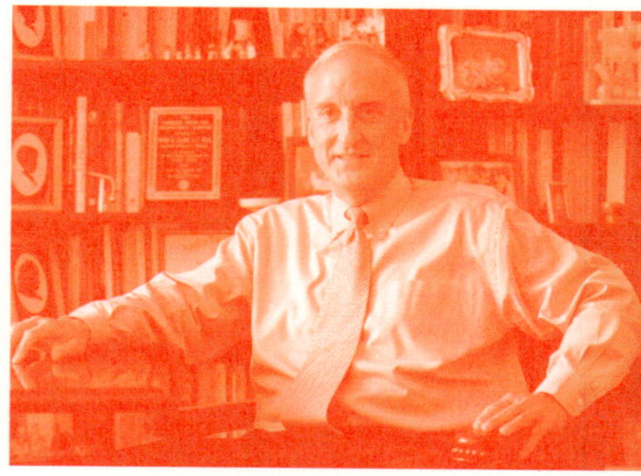
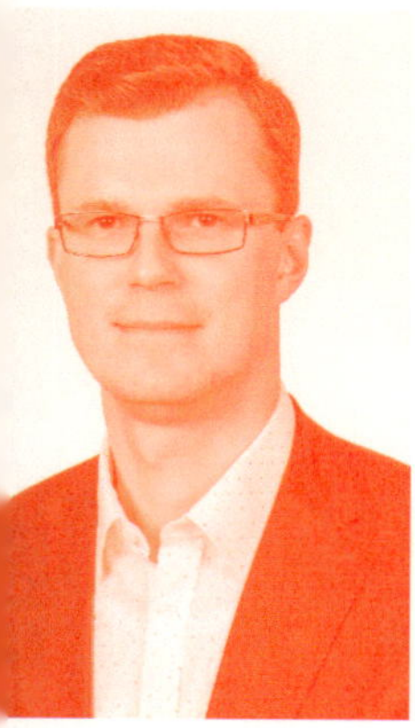
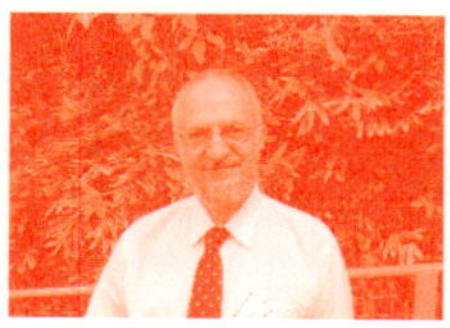
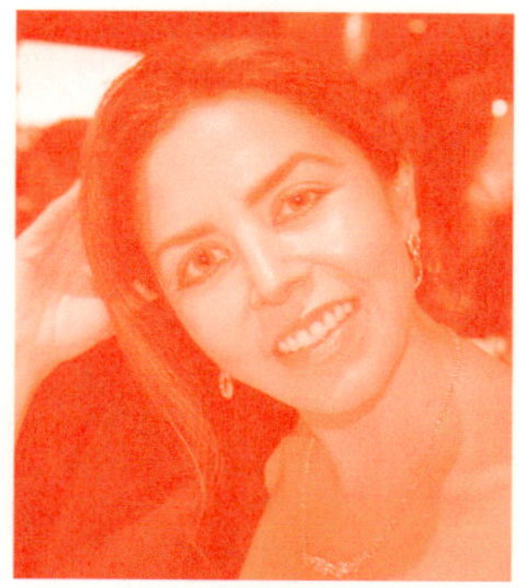

Supporting open minds since 2005

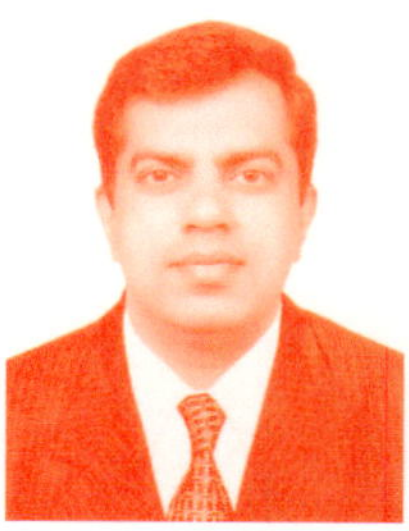
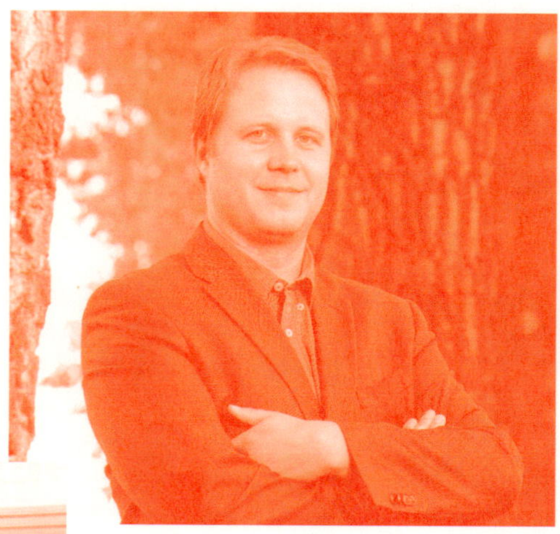
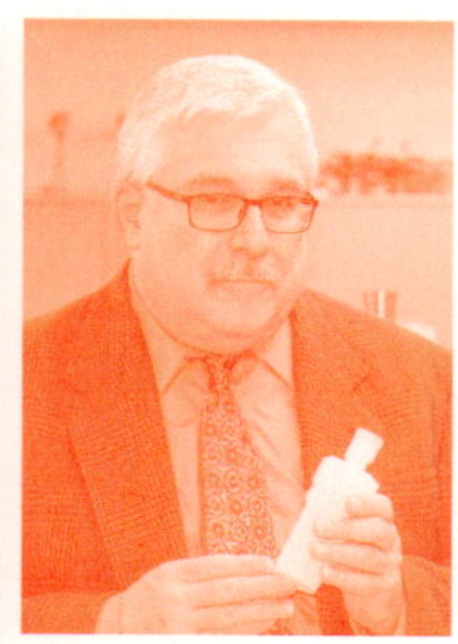
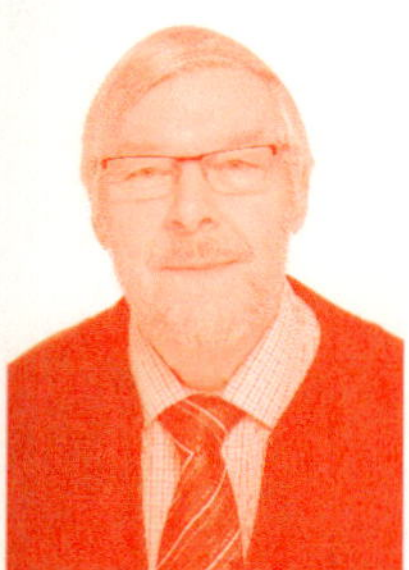
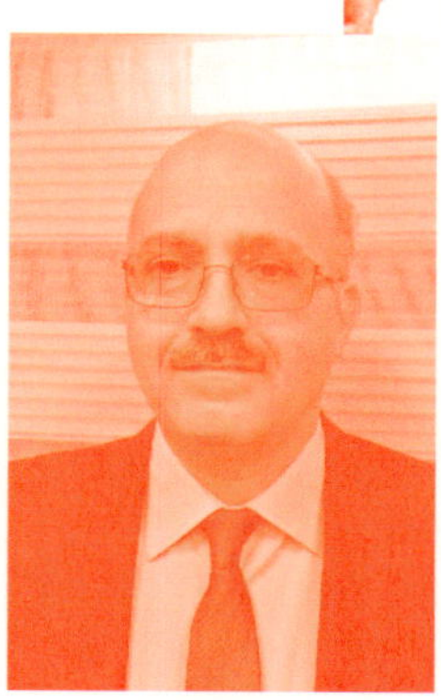
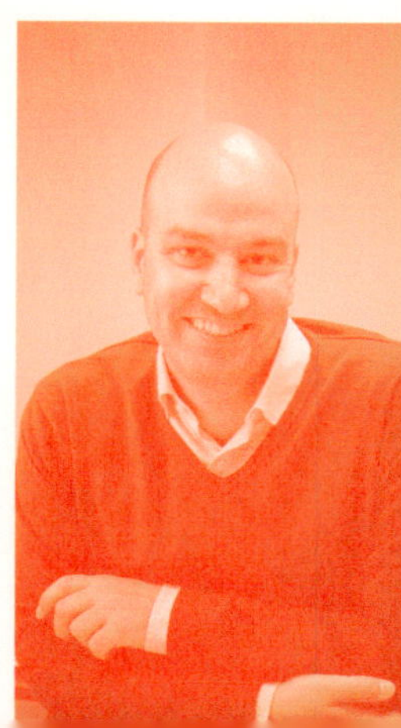
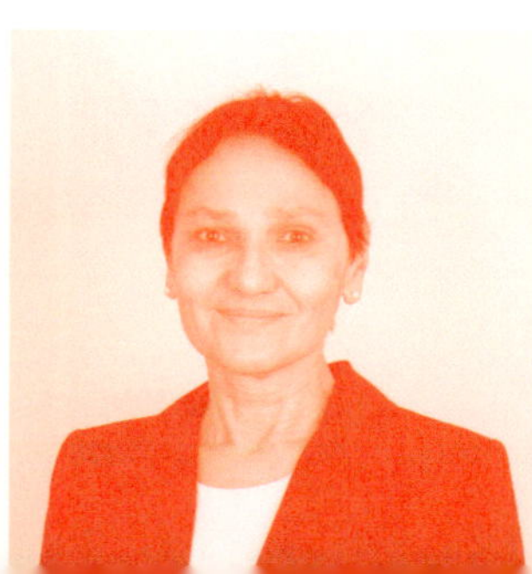

Lower Urinary Tract Dysfunction - From Evidence to Clinical Practice
http://dx.doi.org/10.5772/intechopen.77787
Edited by Ran Pang

Contributors
Francisco Martins, Pedro Simoes De Oliveira, Goran Mitulović, Marianne Koch, Thomas Mohr, Priyanka Bhadana, Charalampos Konstantinidis, Achilleas Karafotias, Ioannis Eleftheropoulos, Bingying Zhou, Jianxin Lu, Peiqi Shi, Yifang An, George Asafu Adjaye Frimpong, Evans Aboagye, Akosua Asafu-Adjaye Frimpong, Ran Pang

First published in London, United Kingdom, 2020 by IntechOpen
IntechOpen is the global imprint of INTECHOPEN LIMITED, registered in England and Wales, registration number: 11086078, 7th floor, 10 Lower Thames Street, London, EC3R 6AF, United Kingdom
Printed in Croatia

British Library Cataloguing-in-Publication Data
A catalogue record for this book is available from the British Library

Additional hard and PDF copies can be obtained from orders@intechopen.com

Lower Urinary Tract Dysfunction - From Evidence to Clinical Practice
Edited by Ran Pang
p. cm.
Print ISBN 978-1-78984-724-6
Online ISBN 978-1-78984-725-3
eBook (PDF) ISBN 978-1-78984-171-8

For EU product safety concerns:
IN TECH d.o.o., Prolaz Marije Krucifikse Kozulić 3, 51000 Rijeka, Croatia, info@intechopen.com or visit our website at intechopen.com.

Meet the editor

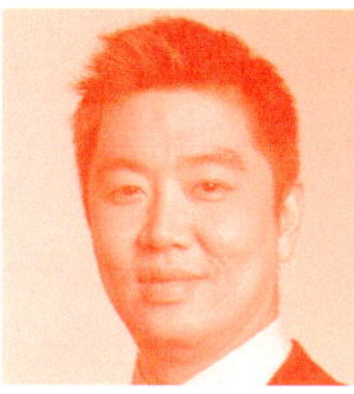

Ran Pang is a consultant urologist and lead in functional urology, and urodynamics at Guang'anmen Hospital, China Academy of Chinese Medical Sciences. After completing residency training, he was accepted to a clinical fellowship with Peking University. Subsequently, he joined a research fellowship at Mayo Clinic, USA, and an urodynamic fellowship in Dalhousie University, Canada. As a leading expert, Dr Pang has published over 40 papers and authored 12 chapters. Moreover, he serves on over 20 academic organizations, such as chair of publication and communication committee, International Continence Society, and vice chair of Pelvic Floor Disorder Group of Urology Committee, Chinese Association of Integrative Medicine. Additionally, he was nominated as a winner of the Albert Nelson Lifetime Achievement award in 2017.

Contents

Preface

Lower urinary tract dysfunction (LUTD) is an umbrella diagnosis that covers the abnormalities of anatomy and function in the bladder, urethra, and, in men, the prostate. People with LUTD face a number of social, mental, and physical health effects due to the symptoms. Despite the increasing evidence in the assessment and management of lower urinary tract symptoms (LUTS), it remains a challenge to bridge the gap between research evidence and clinical practice. In this book, the authors demonstrate their understanding of how to apply the evidence to clinical practice from different aspects.

Based on epidemiological evidence, LUTS are heterogeneous between men and women, which is ascribed to the anatomical difference in the urethra between genders. Generally, pelvic organ prolapse (POP) is a common cause for elderly women to experience LUTS, while benign prostatic hyperplasia is the common cause for elderly men. Accurate evaluation and classification of POP is an important part of physical examination, which is certainly helpful for the development of a therapeutic strategy. Dr Priyanka Bhadana illustrates the assessment approaches of POP. This chapter includes many pictures that will help the readers understand POP.

Besides physical examination, urodynamic study has been playing an important role in the accurate assessment of LUTD. However, the majority of patients tend to prefer a noninvasive assessment compared to invasive urodynamics. Dr George Asafu Adjaye Frimpong and his colleagues present the infeasibility in using imaging modalities, including MRI, CT scan, ultrasound, PET, and fMRI, to assess the function of the lower urinary tract, instead of urodynamics. Not only are the innovative imaging techniques introduced, but also the advantages of each imaging modality for diagnosis of LUTD is interpreted in detail. Although these imaging modalities may not replace urodynamics completely, these approaches can be a substitute for urodynamics and provide useful information for clinicians.

Stress urinary incontinence (SUI) is one of the most common storage LUTS in females. Although the mid-urethral sling results in therapeutic success, it is still unclear how to predict the risk of SUI for individuals. Goran Mitulović introduces an innovative approach to detect potential SUI using proteomic analysis of the urine protein. Once a specific population group susceptible to SUI is identified, active surveillance could be provided as early as possible. In addition, behavior therapy, pelvic floor muscle training, and biofeedback, as a prevention strategy, may also be considered.

Nocturnal enuresis (NE) is a common condition in children. In general, the pathogenesis of NE mainly includes nocturnal polyuria, bladder capacity decline during nighttime, and arousal disorder. With the development of pharmacotherapy, a number of medications can be used to solve these problems. However, how to accurately assess and achieve precision medicine for each patient is still not easy. To help readers develop a proper therapeutic strategy for children with NE, Dr Zhou and her colleagues present current evidence in management of NE. Besides modern medicine, the complementary and alternative medicine approaches are also introduced. It is worth mentioning that Dr Zhou *et al.* show their research results in the chapter, which demonstrates the high level of evidence in the effectiveness of acupuncture in managing NE.

Urethral stricture is a common cause for men to experience lower urinary tract obstruction. Basically, the male urethra consists of the prostatic, membranous, bulbar, and penile urethra. In comparison with other segments, the penile urethral stricture is more complex to reconstruct. Prof. Martins uses a chapter to sketch out an overall perspective on penile urethroplasty. In it, he demonstrates both historical and innovative surgical procedures, which allows readers to obtain an outline of the surgery. Furthermore, he presents an algorithm of surgical reconstruction for different stricture sites, which provides a practical guide for clinicians.

Comorbidity has been the focus in the intervention studies for LUTS. Some recent surveys show a strong association between LUTS and male sexual dysfunction. Understanding the relationship may allow physicians to manage LUTS and sexual dysfunction simultaneously. Dr Konstantinidis and his colleagues bring us a chapter that discusses the comorbidity in the male population. Not only are the involved biochemical pathways described, but the therapeutic strategy is discussed based on current evidence.

In this book, experts and researchers from different countries present the latest evidence in diagnosis and treatment of LUTD. Although these chapters cannot cover all aspects of LUTD, they provide readers with important updates on LUTD. I believe that the more the doctors understand an disease, the more benefit the patients receive. This book is a key to help readers to open the door to LUTD. I hope the book can meet every reader's need.

Ran Pang
Department of Urology,
Guang'anmen Hospital,
China Academy of Chinese Medical Sciences,
Beijing, China

Section 1

Introduction

Chapter 1

Introductory Chapter: Lower Urinary Tract Dysfunction at a Glance

Ran Pang

1. Introduction

Lower urinary tract symptoms (LUTS) refer to a series of symptoms due to bladder or urethral dysfunction and are basically divided into three groups: storage, voiding, and post-micturition symptoms [1]. Of those, storage symptoms include urinary urgency, increased daytime frequency, nocturia, and different types of urinary incontinence. Voiding symptoms include slow stream, splitting or spraying of the urine stream, intermittency, hesitancy, straining to void, and terminal dribble. Post-micturition symptoms include feeling of incomplete emptying and post-micturition dribble. A number of epidemiological studies reported the prevalence of LUTS that varies from country to country. EPIC study performed a population-based, cross-sectional survey in Canada, Germany, Italy, Sweden, and the United Kingdom using computer-assisted telephone interview and showed the overall prevalence of LUTS was approximate 64.3% [2]. The EpiLUTS study investigated the prevalence of LUTS in the USA, United Kingdom, and Sweden according to an Internet-based survey. The results revealed that the prevalence of at least one LUTS in male and female population was 72.3 and 76.3%, respectively [3]. Another study demonstrated that the prevalence in South Korea was 68.5%, which is higher than 59% in Mainland China and 58.5% in Taiwan [4]. The heterogeneity in LUTS prevalence may derive from the difference in genetic, diet, and lifestyle factors for people in different countries. In terms of the gender difference, some studies showed that storage LUTS were more common in women than in men, while voiding and post-micturition LUTS were more common in men than in women [3, 4]. Furthermore, women have a higher proportion to experience storage and voiding LUTS simultaneously in comparison with men. The difference in LUTS between male and female may result from the different anatomy of urethra. Men have an additional organ, prostate, and a longer urethra compared to women, which means men are more likely to experience bladder outlet obstruction than women. Due to the gender difference, it appears to be reasonable to only focus on single-gender population when designing a clinical trial or research about LUTS. Recently a number of clinical trials and research studies have emerged in the assessment and management of LUTS. With the evidence increasing, it is worth considering how to apply these findings to clinical practice. We try to introduce the emerged evidence based on clinical practice from different aspects.

2. Clinical assessment for LUTS

It remains a challenge how to make an accurate assessment for LUTS and identify the potential causes since the etiology of LUTS is diverse. According to EAU guideline, a number of conditions, including detrusor overactivity, underactive bladder, nocturnal polyuria, urethral stricture, etc., may contribute to male LUTS besides benign prostatic obstruction [5]. For female LUTS, increasing evidence shows that bladder outlet obstruction may play an important role in addition to pelvic floor dysfunction [6].

In general, physical examination can provide the helpful information for the etiological diagnosis of LUTS. Besides regular ones, bulbocavernosus reflex test is really useful to check the intactness of S2–S4 spinal reflex arc. Because sacral micturition center is located in S2–S4, this test is helpful to recognize the LUTS secondary to sacral or pudendal neuropathy. Additionally, the evaluation for pelvic floor function is essential for women with LUTS since it can identify the pelvic floor muscle tone, as well as the pelvic organ prolapse.

Traditionally, urodynamic study has been considered as a standard diagnostic tool for lower urinary tract dysfunction. Basically, urodynamic test contains filling cystometry (CMG) and pressure-flow studies (PFSs). The former is used to assess the storage function of the lower urinary tract, whereas the latter is used to evaluate the voiding function. Besides detecting bladder sensitivity, compliance, and detrusor overactivity, CMG can distinguish stress and urgency urinary incontinence. PFSs are normally used to diagnose bladder outlet obstruction. Furthermore, PFSs can also evaluate detrusor contraction, which is useful to find underactive bladder, a common cause of LUTS.

Despite advantages of urodynamic study, majority of patients tend to accept a noninvasive assessment compared to invasive urodynamic test. With the emergence of innovative imaging techniques, both anatomy and function of lower urinary tract can be assessed by noninvasive imaging approaches. In general, ultrasound is the most common technique to diagnose the lower urinary tract dysfunction. Some studies have shown that increased resistance of bladder contraction during the voiding phase in patients with bladder outlet obstruction (BOO) can result in an increase of bladder wall thickness (BWT), so can frequent detrusor overactive (DO) during the storage phase in patients with overactive bladder (OAB) [7, 8]. Based on this finding, a series of ultrasonographic parameters, including BWT, detrusor wall thickness (DWT), and ultrasound-estimated bladder weight (UEBW), have been used to diagnose BOO and DO. Furthermore, ultrasound strain imaging is also a successful method to evaluate LUTS since it can monitor the change in the BWT during micturition in real time. In addition, near-infrared spectroscopy is a functional imaging technique which can detect changes in the concentration of oxygenated hemoglobin and deoxygenated hemoglobin in the bladder wall and consequently identify the DO and BOO. In comparison with ultrasound, MRI may provide additional important clue for the diagnosis of lower urinary tract dysfunction. Brain functional MRI is helpful to detect the neurologic lesions demerging bladder control. Dynamic MRI is able to detect the pelvic organ prolapse, as well as the urethral hypermobility, which cannot be found by physical examination or static MRI.

3. Management of LUTS

Successful management for LUTS is based on the deep understanding on specific symptoms and accurate diagnosis on potential cause of LUTS. For patients with predominant voiding LUTS, it is essential to distinguish between BOO and underactive bladder (UAB). Once BOO is diagnosed clearly, α-blockers could be considered as the initial treatment. For male patients, if the BOO is secondary to significant enlarged prostate (>40 ml), 5α-reductase inhibitor is recommended to be added to shrink the prostate volume [5]. Moreover, there is increasing evidence to suggest phosphodiesterase type 5 inhibitors (PDE5-Is) can relieve LUTS secondary to benign prostatic obstruction effectively though nitric oxide/cyclic guanosine monophosphate pathway (NO/cGMP). For patients who fail to respond to pharmacotherapy, minimal invasive surgical intervention, such as transurethral resection, could be an optional treatment. It is worth mentioning that urethral stricture is also a common cause of BOO and can be treated by urethral dilatation, internal urethrotomy, or urethroplasty depending on the characteristics of the stricture. The management of UAB, by contrast, is controversial because no regulatory approved specific therapy is available so far. Currently, the potential optional treatments for UAB include muscarinic agonists, regenerative therapy with mesenchymal stem cells or autologous muscle derived cells, gene therapy with myoblast injection, and neuromodulation [9].

In terms of patients with predominant storage LUTS, OAB is the most common condition. Although behavioral interventions are recommended to be first-line treatment for OAB by guidelines, muscarinic antagonists and β3 agonists are normally used as the initial treatment in clinical practice. Once pharmacotherapy is unable to improve LUTS effectively, some invasive approaches including sacral neuromodulation, botulinum toxin type A intradetrusor injection, and posterior tibial nerve stimulation can be considered as the advanced therapeutic strategy. Urinary incontinence (UI) is another condition related to storage LUTS, and successful management mainly relies on the precise identification for different types. Urgency UI can be managed by the approaches similar with the ones for OAB. Mid-urethral sling has been mainstream intervention for stress UI since the consolidated theory was proposed by Dr. DeLancey in 1996. Compared to pure stress or urgency UI, mixed UI is more difficult to treat since its complex etiology. Today, the treatment only focuses on the main component of mixed UI. Besides conventional therapy, increasing high-level evidence demonstrates the effectiveness of complementary and alternative medicine on different types of UI [10, 11]. Nocturia is also a bothersome storage LUTS which not only can weaken patients' quality of life but also may increase the risk of mortality. Management of nocturia had been a controversial issue until the classification of nocturia was proposed, which allows clinicians to provide precision treatment for patients. It is reported that the main factors contributing to nocturia include nocturnal polyuria and bladder capacity decline during nighttime. The former can be managed by desmopressin or diuretics, whereas the latter can be treated by muscarinic antagonists and β3 agonists. It is important to differentiate nocturnal enuresis from nocturia in clinical practice, because both of them occur during the nighttime. The main difference between the two symptoms is whether the patient is accompanied by sleep arousal. Nocturnal enuresis occurs during sleep, while nocturia is presented in arousal. Moreover, nocturnal enuresis, also known as bed-wetting, is more likely to present in children, while nocturia is common in adults. Similar to the pathogenesis of nocturia, nocturnal polyuria, and bladder capacity decline during nighttime are the potential pathogenesis of nocturnal enuresis too. Besides, arousal disorder also plays an important role for the occurrence of nocturnal enuresis. For this factor, alarm therapy could be helpful in waking the children up.

In summary, accurate clinical assessment is the prerequisite to manage LUTS successfully. Only with the sufficient understanding in characteristics and potential causes of LUTS can an individual management strategy be developed, which may optimize the treatment effect.

Acknowledgements

This work was supported by Beijing Municipal Science and Technology Commission No. Z161100000516156 and grant 2014S292 from Guang'anmen Hospital, China Academy of Chinese Medical Sciences.

Author details

Ran Pang
Guang'anmen Hospital, China Academy of Chinese Medical Sciences, Beijing, China

*Address all correspondence to: pangran2002@gmail.com

References

[1] Abrams P et al. The standardisation of terminology of lower urinary tract function: Report from the Standardisation Sub-committee of the International Continence Society. Neurourology and Urodynamics. 2002;**21**(2):167-178

[2] Irwin DE et al. Population-based survey of urinary incontinence, overactive bladder, and other lower urinary tract symptoms in five countries: Results of the EPIC study. European Urology. 2006;**50**(6):1306-1314; discussion 1314-5

[3] Coyne KS et al. The prevalence of lower urinary tract symptoms (LUTS) in the USA, the UK and Sweden: Results from the epidemiology of LUTS (EpiLUTS) study. BJU International. 2009;**104**(3):352-360

[4] Chapple C et al. Prevalence of lower urinary tract symptoms in China, Taiwan, and South Korea: Results from a cross-sectional, population-based study. Advances in Therapy. 2017;**34**(8):1953-1965

[5] Gratzke C et al. EAU guidelines on the assessment of non-neurogenic male lower urinary tract symptoms including benign prostatic obstruction. European Urology. 2015;**67**(6):1099-1109

[6] Malde S et al. Female bladder outlet obstruction: Common symptoms masking an uncommon cause. Lower Urinary Tract Symptoms. 2019;**11**(1):72-77

[7] Kuo HC. Measurement of detrusor wall thickness in women with overactive bladder by transvaginal and transabdominal sonography. International Urogynecology Journal and Pelvic Floor Dysfunction. 2009;**20**(11):1293-1299

[8] Robinson D et al. Can ultrasound replace ambulatory urodynamics when investigating women with irritative urinary symptoms? BJOG. 2002;**109**(2):145-148

[9] Chai TC, Kudze T. New therapeutic directions to treat underactive bladder. Investigative and Clinical Urology. 2017;**58**(Suppl 2):S99-S106

[10] Liu B et al. Electroacupuncture versus pelvic floor muscle training plus solifenacin for women with mixed urinary incontinence: A randomized noninferiority trial. Mayo Clinic Proceedings. 2019;**94**(1):54-65

[11] Liu Z et al. Effect of electroacupuncture on urinary leakage among women with stress urinary incontinence: A randomized clinical trial. JAMA. 2017;**317**(24):2493-2501

Section 2

Assessment

Chapter 2

Pelvic Organ Prolapse: Examination and Assessment

Priyanka Bhadana

Abstract

Pelvic organ prolapse (POP) is a common, benign condition in women, and patient can present with complaints of vaginal bulge and pressure, voiding and defecatory, and sexual dysfunction, which may adversely affect quality of life. Although POP can occur in younger women, it is commonly seen in aging population with a prevalence of 45–50%. Older terms describing pelvic organ prolapse (e.g., cystocele, urethrocele, rectocele) have been replaced because they do not provide complete information regarding the structures on the other side of the vaginal bulge, especially in women who have had previous pelvic organ prolapse surgery. Therefore, a thorough history and performing a careful physical examination with dignity and care, using some basic tools that aid in the accurate evaluation of anatomical and functional defects, should be conducted. A standardized assessment system has been used to document findings which should explain everything in understandable terms.

Keywords: uterovaginal prolapse, POP-Q

1. Introduction

Pelvic organ prolapse (POP) is the herniation of the pelvic organs to or beyond the vaginal walls. Many women with prolapse experience symptoms that impact daily activities, sexual function, and exercise. The presence of POP can have a detrimental impact on body image and sexuality. Pelvic organ prolapse is an increasingly common condition seen with aging population with a prevalence of 41–50% of women above 40 years. The annual incidence of surgery for POP is within the range of 15–49 cases per 10,000 women years [1]. Pelvic floor defects result from attenuation of the supportive structures or by neuromuscular dysfunction due to obstetric trauma. Pregnancy itself, without vaginal birth, has been cited as a risk factor as well. Genital atrophy and hypoestrogenism also play important contributory roles in the pathogenesis of prolapse. However, the exact mechanisms are not completely understood. Prolapse may potentially result from pelvic tumors, sacral nerve disorders, and diabetic neuropathy [2].

Older terms describing pelvic organ prolapse (e.g., cystocele, urethrocele, rectocele) have been replaced because they do not provide complete information regarding the structures on the other side of the vaginal bulge, especially in women who have had previous pelvic organ prolapse surgery.

Presently, the pelvis is divided into anterior, posterior, and middle or apical compartments. Following hysterectomy, prolapse of the vaginal apex with or without prolapse of the anterior and/or posterior vaginal wall is referred to as vault prolapse [2, 3].

2. Classification of pelvic organ prolapse

Pelvic organ support is maintained by complex interactions between the vagina, levator ani muscle, and pelvic floor connective tissue. A system of three integrated levels of vaginal support has been described by De Lancey [1].

- Level 1: The cardinal uterosacral ligament complex.
- Level 2: Midvaginal supports—pubocervical and rectovaginal fascia.
- Level 3: Urogenital diaphragm and the perineal body.

The prolapse is usually described according to the area of the vagina in which it occurs. Assumptions are often made about which organ is behind the vaginal wall that is prolapsing.

Anatomical classification according to vaginal wall:

- Anterior: cystocele (bladder most common) and urethrocele (urethra).
- Middle: vault of the uterus (after hysterectomy).
- Posterior: rectocele (rectum) and enterocele (small bowel, omentum).

2.1 Shaw's classification

- Anterior wall
    - Upper 2/3 cystocele
    - Lower 1/3 urethrocele
- Posterior wall
    - Upper 1/3 enterocele
    - Middle 1/3 rectocele
    - Lower 1/3 deficient perineum
- Uterine prolapse
    - Grade 0: Normal position
    - Grade 1: Descent into vagina not reaching the introitus

- Grade 2: Descent up to the introitus
- Grade 3: Descent outside the introitus
- Grade 4: Procidentia [2]

- Uterovaginal prolapse usually occurs in nulliparous prolapse due to congenital weakness of cervical ligaments.
- Vaginouterine prolapse usually occurs in cases of prolapse resulting from obstetrical trauma.

3. Pelvic organ prolapse quantification system (POP-Q)

Pelvic organ prolapse quantification system refers to an objective, site-specific system for describing, quantifying, and staging pelvic support in women (**Figure 1**). It provides a standardized tool for documenting, comparing, and communicating clinical findings with proven interobserver and intraobserver reliability. The POP-Q system gained the attention of the specialists all over the world, being approved by the International Continence Society (ICS), the American Urogynecologic Society (AUGS), and the Society of Gynecologic Surgeons for the description of female pelvic organ prolapse. It is the most common system used by gynecologists and urogynecologists, although other systems have been devised (**Figures 2–9**) [4].

The POP-Q may be an easier classification system to use in routine clinical practice. It was developed by the International Urogynecological Association to provide a less cumbersome exam tool [4]. The POP-Q stages (**Table 1**) prolapse

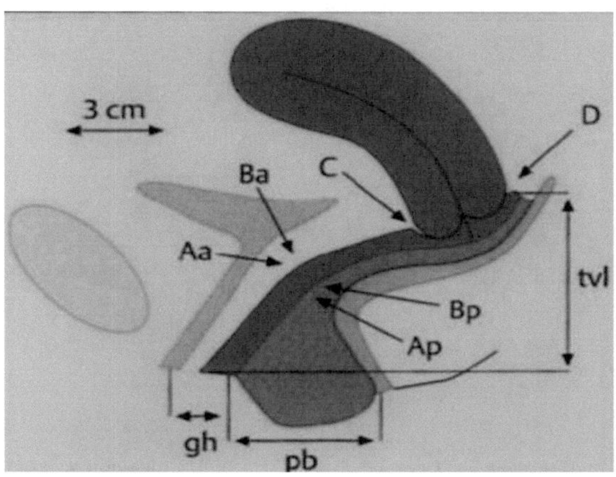

Figure 1.
POP-Q points. Aa, anterior vaginal wall 3 cm proximal to the urethral meatus (−3 cm to +3 cm); Ba,most distal position of the remaining upper anterior vaginal wall (−3 cm to +tvl); C, most distal edge of cervix or vaginal cuff scar; D, posterior fornix (n/a if posthysterectomy); Ap, posterior vaginal wall 3 cm proximal to the hymen (−3 cm to +3 cm); Bp, most distal position of the remaining upper posterior vaginal wall (−3 cm to + tvl); genital hiatus (gh), measured from the middle of external urethral meatus to the posterior midline hymen; perineal body (pb), measured from the posterior margin of gh to the middle of anal opening; total vaginal length (tvl), depth of the vagina when point D or C is reduced to normal position.

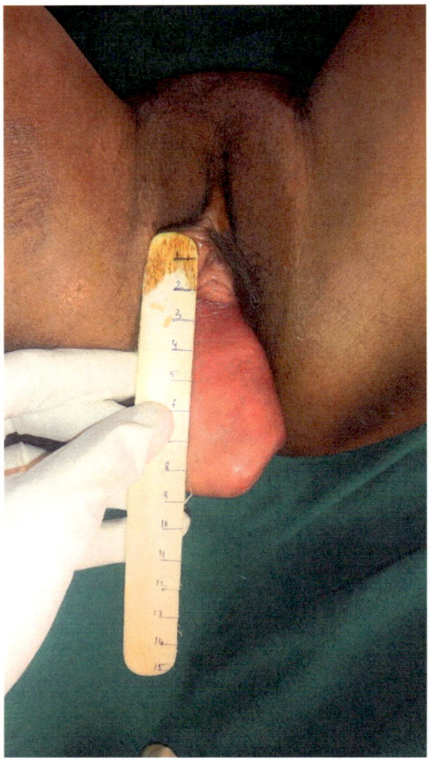

Figure 2.
Point Aa being measured by graded spatula.

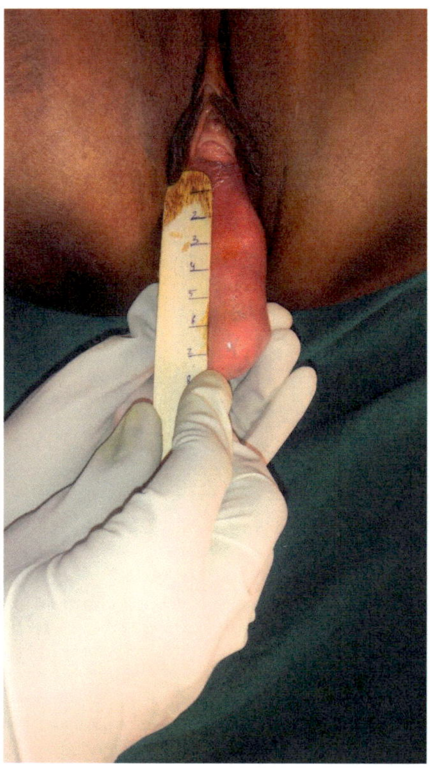

Figure 3.
Point Ba being measured by graded spatula.

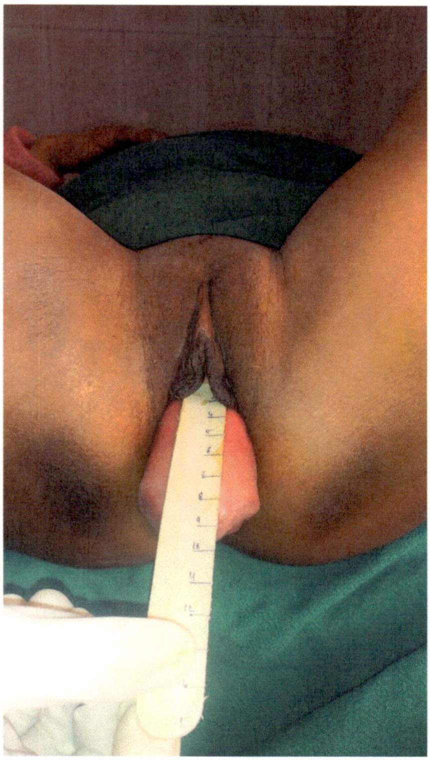

Figure 4.
Point C.

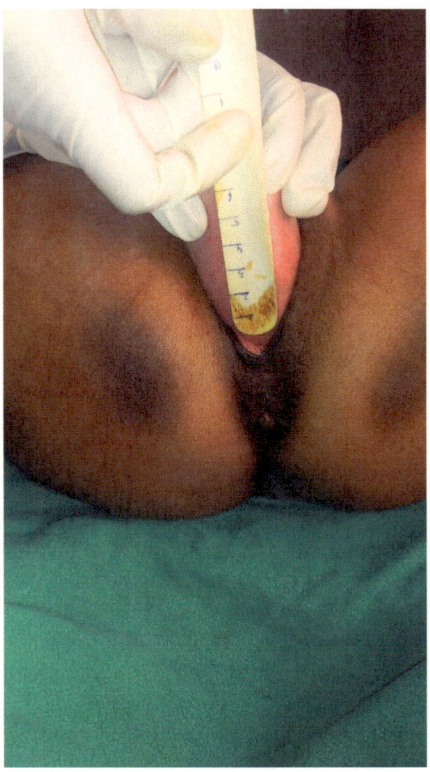

Figure 5.
Point Ap.

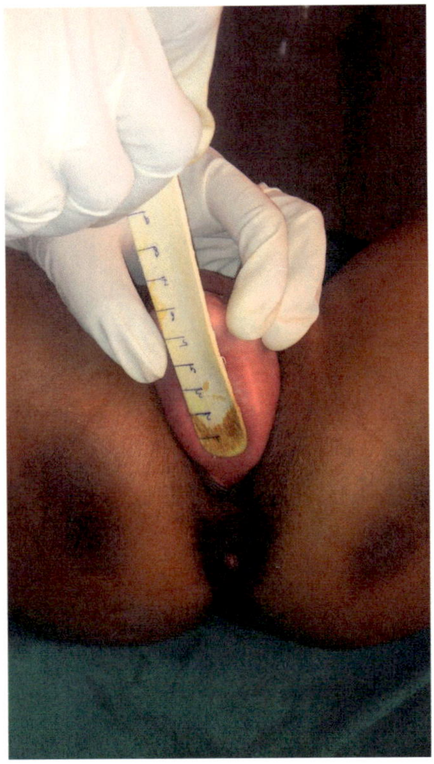

Figure 6.
Point Bp.

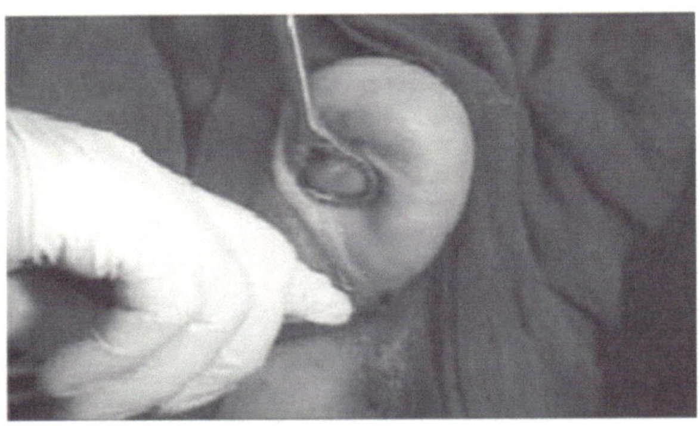

Figure 7.
Point D.

for the anterior and posterior vaginal walls, the apex/cuff of the vagina and the cervix. For women posthysterectomy, there are three stages; for women with an intact uterus, there are four. The exam is carried out similarly to the standard POP-Q exam, with a half speculum placed in the vagina to visualize the vaginal walls and cervix.

A disadvantage of POP-Q is that all points and measures are taken in the midline; as a consequence, the POP-Q does not reflect asymmetries and cannot be used to describe, for example, paravaginal defects. One has also to keep in mind that the POP-Q depends on the cooperation of the patient and to the strength of her cough or Valsalva maneuver; it is therefore unreasonable to assume that in an individual patient, the POP-Q will always be identical [4].

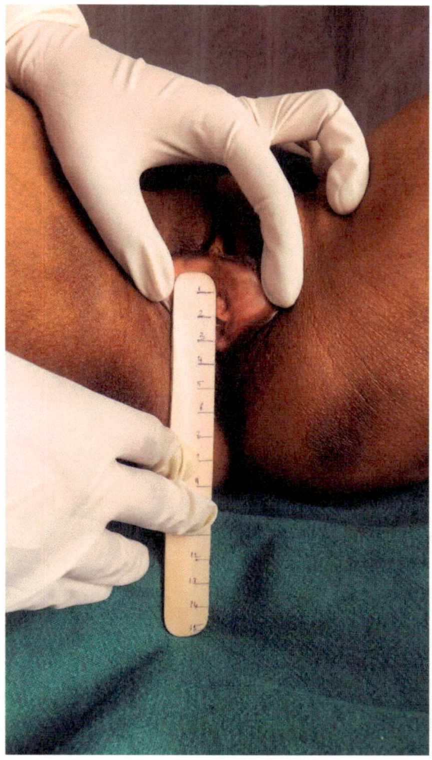

Figure 8.
Genital hiatus (gh).

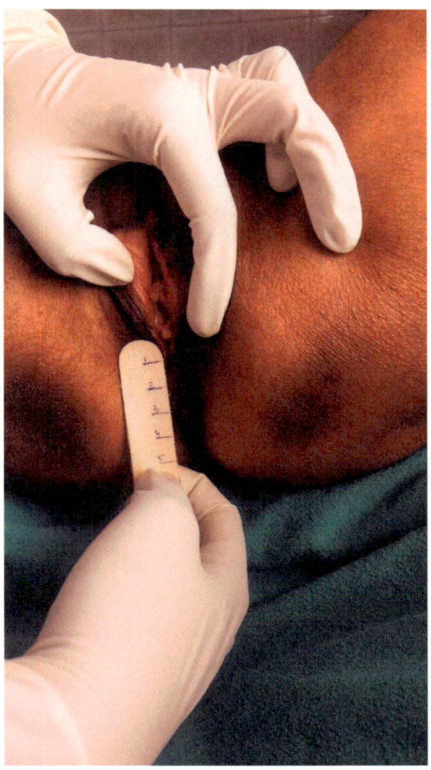

Figure 9.
Perineal body (P_b).

Pelvic organ prolapse quantification system	
Stage	**Description**
0	No prolapse
I	>1 cm above the hymen
II	≤1 cm proximal or distal to the plane of the hymen
III	>1 cm below the plane of the hymen, but protrudes no farther than 2 cm less than the total vaginal length
IV	Eversion of the lower genital tract is complete

POP-Q staging criteria.
Stage 0: Aa, Ap, Ba, Bp = −3 cm and C or D ≤ − (tvl − 2) cm.
Stage l: Stage 0 criteria not met and leading edge < −1 cm.
Stage ll: Leading edge ≥ −1 cm but ≤ +1 cm.
Stage lll: Leading edge > +1 cm but < + (tvl − 2) cm.
Stage lV: Leading edge ≥ + (tvl −2) cm [3, 4].

Table 1.
Evaluation/staging of pelvic organ prolapse.

4. History

Most patients with pelvic organ prolapse are asymptomatic. Seeing or feeling a bulge of tissue that protrudes to or past the vaginal opening is the most specific symptom.

4.1 Bulge in the vagina

During a well-woman examination, she should be asked regarding any obvious bulge seen or felt in vagina. The report of a bulge has an 81% positive predictive value and a 76% negative predictive value for pelvic organ prolapse.

Patient may complain of an increase in bulging and discomfort with progression of day [1]. Extensive standing, lifting, coughing, and physical exertion may increase patient awareness of discomfort in the pelvis, vagina, abdomen, and low back. Pelvic organ prolapse may progress with increasing body mass index. Weight loss does not reverse the prolapse.

4.2 Vaginal discharge

Vaginal discharge may be present in patients with complete uterine prolapse (i.e., procidentia) who have a decubitus ulcer of the cervix or vagina.

4.3 Urinary symptoms

Patients may have difficulty urinating—stress incontinence affects 40% of patients with pelvic organ prolapse; therefore, they should be asked about frequency, urgency, and sensation of incomplete emptying of the bladder, because they may not volunteer such information. Urinary outlet obstruction may occur because of the pressure on the urethra in anterior vaginal prolapse and sometimes in large posterior vaginal prolapse. Screening is advocated for urinary tract infection, postvoid residual urine volume, and the presence or absence of bladder sensation.

Symptoms may not correlate with the location or severity of the prolapsed compartment.

4.4 Bowel symptoms

Patients with posterior vaginal prolapse sometimes use manual pressure on the perineum or posterior vagina to help with defecation. These maneuvers are called "splinting."

4.5 Back pain

Though patients of prolapse attribute back and pelvic pain to their prolapse, very little evidence is available to show that this disorder causes pain, so other causes of pain should be ruled out.

4.6 Sexual discomfort

Sexual activity, body image, and quality of life may be affected [3].

5. Examination

5.1 General physical examination

Assessment will include weight, body mass index, and blood pressure, as well as assessment of any varicose veins or hypermobile joints, since these can be markers of a tendency to connective tissue laxity which predisposes to POP and, importantly, to recurrence after surgical repair [2].

5.2 Abdominal examination

On examination of the abdomen, inspect for incisions of previous surgery (which may be associated with intra-abdominal adhesions affecting subsequent surgical approaches), and exclude masses or ascites. The presence of umbilical or other hernia can again indicate underlying connective tissue weakness and may require concomitant surgical correction [2, 3].

5.3 Local examination

On inspection of the vulva, note the presence of any atrophy and whether there is any ulceration of prolapsed tissues that may require local estrogen therapy before surgery. Wide genital hiatus with visible vaginal walls or midline asymmetry on Valsalva shows levator ani damage.

For stress urinary incontinence, the patient needs to be examined with full bladder and asked to cough or strain, and leakage of urine confirms positive stress provocation test.

On examination in lithotomy position, if there is visible vaginal bulge, look for vaginal wall rugosities which predict an intact fascial layer in the midline and a probable lateral defect, or if absent, it suggests a midline defect with only the skin and attenuated connective tissue present.

6. Examination in various positions

6.1 Standing position

In some mild cases of vaginal wall and uterine prolapse, examination of the patient in standing position is the only way to explore it.

6.2 Dorsal position

Mostly for demonstration of uterine prolapse. Either the uterus will be obviously protruded or protrude when the patient is asked to strain.

6.3 Sims' position

In this position, the aim is to demonstrate the different types of vaginal wall prolapse. The patient is asked to lie on her left side at the edge of the table. The left leg is extended, while the right leg is flexed. Afterward, a sterile Sims' speculum is inserted into the vagina gently first to expose the anterior vaginal wall. Then it is pulled backward gradually to expose the posterior vaginal wall. Cystocele and rectocele are usually diagnosed by this examination.

7. Per speculum examination

Examination with a Cusco's bivalve speculum allows assessment of the cervix (including a Pap smear, if appropriate), but not of prolapse. The use of a Sims' speculum is required to carefully assess the anterior and posterior compartments and to assess the supports of the cervix or the vault if there has been a previous hysterectomy. If prolapse is visible at the vaginal introitus or on Valsalva maneuver, a systematic examination should be performed. With the patient in a supine position, a suitable sized vaginal speculum is introduced in the vagina to view the cervix or vaginal cuff, and the extent to which the cervix or the vaginal vault follows the speculum through and out of the vagina is noted, and the speculum is slowly removed while performing Valsalva maneuver.

To examine the anterior vaginal wall, the posterior vaginal wall is retracted with the fixed blade, and the extent of any anterior vaginal prolapse during the Valsalva maneuver is noted and vice versa to examine posterior vaginal wall. Any resulting prolapse is noted.

Decubitus ulcers are inspected and palpated. It is common to require sponge holding forceps to aid in support of the vaginal walls, as this can obscure the view.

8. Per vaginal and rectovaginal examination

Bimanual examination is performed to check the uterine size and mobility, as well as to exclude unsuspected adnexal pathology, such as ovarian tumors. This also allows an assessment of vaginal muscle tone. Rectal examination may distinguish rectocele from enterocele. Make sure you ask the woman to direct your attention to any other findings that she has noted, that you have not discovered, or that she wants to draw your attention to.

Bonney's stress test is performed following reduction of prolapsed. If test is positive, incontinence surgery should be performed at the time of prolapse surgery. Testing for integrity of anal sphincter should be assessed for resting tone and voluntary squeeze and sensation around the vulva with the bulbocavernous reflex. (Stroking lateral to clitoris contraction of bilateral bulbocavernous muscle is observed.) The anocutaneous reflex (anal wink sign) is triggered by stroking the skin immediately surrounding the anus and observing a reflexive contraction of the external anal sphincter; this reflex should be elicited bilaterally. Absence of these reflexes is not always abnormal, and hyperreflexia or asymmetry may in fact be more suggestive of a neurologic etiology. Crude sensory testing is advocated for evidence of pudendal neuropathy [4, 5].

Grading pelvic floor muscle strength:

1. No discernible contraction.

2. Barely palpable, flickering contraction, not visible on inspection of the perineum.

3. Weak, distinctly palpable contraction, felt as slight pressure on the examining finger.

4. Moderate muscle strength, distinct pressure on the examining finger, palpable upward and forward movement, visible on the perineal surface.

5. Good muscle strength, elevation possible against slight resistance, circular pressure can be felt around the examining finger. During simultaneous examination by the index and middle finger, these are pressed against each other.

6. Very strong muscle strength, contraction possible against vigorous resistance, with suction-type effect on the examining finger. During simultaneous examination by the index and middle finger, these are pressed against each other despite resistance.

Digital examination makes it possible to distinguish between the left and right side of the levator ani. It is capable of quantifying strength, strength endurance, fast contraction, and fast contraction endurance for clinical purposes [2].

9. Quantifying and documenting the findings

A full description of the examination is recorded, including the following:

- Type of examination table, speculum, and retractors
- Patient position
- Bladder and rectal fullness

It is important to note and document any episodes of urinary, fecal, or flatal incontinence that occur during the examination. The findings of the examination should be recorded using a quantitative and reproducible method for recording POP such as the POP-Q, Baden-Walker, or Shaw systems [4, 5].

10. Further evaluation

Further studies depend on the symptoms, stage of prolapse, and treatment plan. If needed for definitive treatment planning, urodynamic studies can help in identifying those patients with lower urinary tract symptoms (urinary incontinence) who are most likely to get benefit from surgery or may require stress incontinence surgery. Patients with defecatory symptoms and/or fecal incontinence may need anal manometry and endoanal ultrasonography [5].

11. Conclusion

Taking a thorough history and performing a careful physical examination of women who are referred help in the assessment of prolapse. Examination should be carried out with dignity and care, using some basic tools that aid in the accurate evaluation of anatomical and functional defects. A standardized assessment system has been used to document findings which should explain everything in understandable terms.

Author details

Priyanka Bhadana
ABVIMS and RML Hospital, New Delhi, India

*Address all correspondence to: docpriyanka89@gmail.com

References

[1] Shaw R, Luesley D, Monga A, editors. Urogynaecology Section. Gynaecology, 4th ed. London: Churchill Livingstone; 2010

[2] Bordman R, Telner D, et al. Step-by-step approach to managing pelvic organ prolapse. Can Fam Physician. 2007;**53**(3):485-487

[3] Kuncharapu I, Majeroni BA. Pelvic organ prolapsed Am fam physician. 2010;**81**(9):1111-1117

[4] Kieren W, Andrew F. Prolapse assessment. Int urogynecol J. 2014;**16**(1):35

[5] ACOG Committee on practice bulletins—gynecology. ACOG practice bulletin no. 85: Pelvic organ prolapse. Obstetrics and Gynecology. 2007;**110**(3):717-729

Chapter 3

Diagnostic Potential of Imaging Modalities in the Assessment of Lower Urinary Tract Dysfunctions

George Asafu Adjaye Frimpong, Evans Aboagye and Akosua Asafu-Adjaye Frimpong

Abstract

Lower urinary tract dysfunction (LUTD) is common in both men and women, and the incidence and prevalence increases as people age. Commonly observed symptoms of LUTD include nocturia, urgency, urinary incontinence and frequency of voiding. Recognizing the key role accurate monitoring and evaluation of LUTD play in the day-to-day assessment of the condition, this chapter will explore the diagnostic capabilities of imaging modalities including MRI, ultrasound and fluoroscopy in assessing bladder wall thickness (BWT), detrusor wall thickness (DWT) and estimation of bladder weight both in real-time and static positions, and finally analyze their suitability as surrogates for bladder outlet obstruction (BOO) or detrusor overactivity (DO).

Keywords: lower urinary tract dysfunction, bladder, MRI, ultrasound, PET

1. Introduction

The lower urinary tract (LUT), consisting of the urinary bladder and urethra, functions to store and expel urine in a controlled and coordinated manner [1, 2]. This key function is dependent upon neural circuits located in the central and peripheral nervous system (CNS) (brain, peripheral ganglia, spinal cord and brain) [1], thus distinguishing LUT from other visceral structures such as cardiovascular system and gastrointestinal tract, that are able to sustain a certain level of activity even after elimination of extrinsic neural input [3]. Considering the fact that control over urine storage and voiding is somehow complex and also dependent on neurological elements widely distributed in anatomical terms, the function of LUT can be affected by a myriad of neurological diseases and disorders of the peripheral organs [4].

Lower urinary tract dysfunctions (LUTD) may thus result from lesions affecting the brain, suprasacral spinal cord and sacral spinal cord or peripheral nerve [5]. Lesions affecting the suprasacral or spinal pathways affect the storage phase, leading to reduced bladder capacity and detrusor overactivity, which is characterized by varying degrees of urinary frequency, urgency, incontinence and nocturia, while lesions of the sacral spinal cord pathways result in voiding dysfunction, associated with non-relaxing sphincter and/or absent or poorly sustained detrusor contractions [6]. As a result, functional disorders such as bladder outlet obstruction secondary to prostatic enlargement, overactive bladder and urinary incontinence are common, as are prostate and bladder carcinoma [7].

Clinical assessment of LUDT may include tests such as post-void residual volume measurement, renal ultrasound, uroflowmetry, urethrocystoscopy, neurophysiology and urodynamics depending on the indication [6]. Furthermore, urodynamic tests including filling cystometry and pressure flow study are considered as the gold standard methods for diagnosing detrusor overactivity (DO) and bladder outlet obstruction (BOO) respectively. The key issue with the urodynamic techniques is that, they are invasive and hence are associated with potential patient morbidity [8]. Therefore, there have been efforts over the years toward developing non-invasive techniques such as ultrasound, magnetic resonance imaging (MRI), fluoroscopy and near-infrared spectroscopy, with the potential of serving as suitable surrogates for diagnosing BOO and DO. Recognizing the key role these imaging modalities play in accurate monitoring and evaluation of LUTD, this chapter set out to explore their diagnostic potential in LUTD and finally examine their suitability as surrogates for the urodynamic tests.

2. The lower urinary tract

The lower urinary tract (LUT) consists of urinary bladder and urethra, and also includes the prostate in males. These organs are actively involved in the involuntary storage of urine formed in the upper urinary tract and the voluntary expulsion of urine at a suitable place and time [7]. The effectiveness of these functions depend on the activity of striated and smooth muscles in the bladder, urethra and external urethral sphincter, which is in turn controlled by neural circuits in the spinal cord, peripheral ganglia and brain [4]. Owning to the differences in sexual function and pelvic anatomy, there are considerable differences in the anatomy of LUT in males and females.

The bladder is a hollow organ located within the pelvis. Its wall consists of five layers from inside out, and the muscle of the bladder, the detrusor, is composed of smooth muscle fibers [9]. The wall thickness of the bladder decreases from 2 cm to 2 mm during expansion. The principal function of the bladder is that of a reservoir, storing urine at lower pressures, even with large filling volumes. The normal bladder holds 200–500 ml urine, and for imaging assessment, a full bladder is preferred for visualization. Due to the visco-elastic properties of the bladder wall and the inhibition of the filling phase detrusor contractions, the bladder is compliant and the pressure inside usually remain low [10]. In the clinical assessment of images of the LUT, it is important to note the close relation between the anterior vaginal wall and the urethra in women and between seminal vesicles and prostate and posterior urethra and the bladder base in men [11].

2.1 Lower urinary tract dysfunction (LUTD)

The primary physiological functions of the LUT are the storage of urine (at relatively low pressure) and its voiding (expulsion) at appropriate time. LUT dysfunction is a common problem, and the prevalence increases with ageing. The term “dysfunction” indicates an abnormality in the physiology of the lower urinary tract, including urinary sphincter, associated nervous system, bladder neck and detrusor muscle. This may result in failure to store urine, failure to empty or a combination of both [12]. Lower urinary tract symptoms can thus be divided into storage phase symptoms, voiding phase symptoms and postmicturition symptoms. These symptoms can be caused by various types of bladder dysfunctions such as overactive bladder, underactive bladder, urinary tract infections and neurogenic disorders [13]. Storage symptoms include increased nocturia, daytime frequency, urgency and incontinence. Voiding symptoms include splitting or spraying, slow stream, intermittency, hesitancy, straining and terminal dribble. Post micturition symptoms include a feeling of incomplete emptying and post micturition dribble [14].

2.1.1 Bladder outlet obstruction (BOO)

Voiding as intended by nature should result in complete emptying of the bladder. This depends on a coordinated contraction of the detrusor smooth muscle with a simultaneous lowering of bladder outlet resistance. Distortion, compression or occlusion of the outlet of the bladder obstructs urine flow during expulsion, with attendant characteristic symptoms of dribbling, poor stream, incomplete emptying and hesitancy. Bladder outlet obstruction (BOO) is an indication of the existence of abnormal tissue which modifies the configuration of the bladder outlet through distortion, compression or occlusion, thus impeding the urine flow at the time of expulsion. Accompanying urine symptoms include slow stream, intermittent stream, hesitancy, straining to void, terminal dribble, post-micturition dribble and feeling of incomplete emptying [15].

These LUT symptoms are caused by a variety of different pathologies. The commonest processes responsible for BOO in men are benign prostatic enlargement (BPE) or urethral stricture disease [15]. For lesser degrees of obstruction, the symptomatic consequences may be slight, owing to compensatory responses, such as enhanced bladder contractility. However, a potential feature of BPE is the progression of obstruction with ageing, which leads to evident expulsion and post-micturition LUT symptoms. Also, the emergence of LUT symptoms point to relative inadequacy in the expulsive capacity of the bladder, which may be a consequence of detrusor underactivity. Detrusor underactivity is characterized by a contraction of reduced duration and/or strength, thus resulting in failure to achieve complete bladder emptying within regular time span and/or prolonged bladder emptying. The variables of detrusor contraction strength, contraction duration and outlet obstruction severity leads to varied clinical features of BOO. The basis of obstruction in females may be bladder neck distortion, urethral compression or luminal occlusion and functional issues [16]. However, in women, due to difficulty in assessing bladder contractility, there is difficulty in arriving at decisions on issues regarding diagnosis of BOO [15]. Diagnosis of BOO can be made based on invasive urodynamic study, such as videourodynamic study or pressure flow study. Also, a noninvasive method to diagnose BOO is needed for more accurate treatment [17].

2.1.2 Overactive bladder (OAB) and detrusor overactivity (DO)

According to the International Continence Society (ICS), overactive bladder (OAB) is defined as a complex of urgency, usually with increased daytime frequency and nocturia, with (OAB wet) or without (OAB dry) urinary incontinence. Urgency is the key symptom of OAB, and it is a sudden compelling desire to pass urine, which is difficult to defer [18]. In diagnosing OAB, it is assumed that conflicting issues such as, urinary tract infections are excluded. OAB might be because of increased bladder sensation or detrusor overactivity (DO). Confusion usually exists between these two disease states because patients usually cannot differentiate the sensation of urgency from the urge to void [19].

DO is an urodynamic observation characterized by involuntary detrusor contractions during the filling phase that may be provoked or spontaneous. The ICS

2002 report categorizes DO into two types: (1) terminal, which is a single involuntary detrusor contraction that often results in complete bladder emptying; and (2) phasic, which may or may not lead to urinary incontinence. Therefore, OAB is a symptom-based diagnosis, while DO is an urodynamic diagnosis. A research on OAB and DOO showed that 64% of patients with OAB symptoms had DO on urodynamic investigation, while 30% of the patients with DO did not have AOB [18].

3. Imaging modalities used for the clinical assessment of LUTD

The lower urinary tract (LUT) requires coordination of the prostate, bladder, pelvic floor, urethra, and specific spinal cord and brain areas. Different imaging modalities can be utilized to visualize these structures and are employed to study its pathophysiology and diagnose voiding dysfunction. Although the bladder and urethra are anatomically distinct structures, they are functionally closely interrelated. Therefore, imaging of the bladder is often needed to confirm clinical examination.

Imaging modalities including ultrasound (US), voiding cystourethrogram X-ray (VCUG), magnetic resonance imaging (MRI), computed tomography (CT), positron emission tomography (PET) and functional magnetic resonance imaging (fMRI) are used to visualize the distinctive structures of the LUT. US is the commonly used technique in daily practice, to evaluate LUTD. The utilization of MRI for voiding dysfunction however remains limited, but several clinical studies have already shown its potential in the benign prostatic hyperplasia (BPH) and diagnosis of stress urinary incontinence. Also, PET and fMRI of the brain have made it possible to study supraspinal control of the LUT, in the light of LUT being subjected to a complex neural control mechanism.

Urodynamic tests have over the years been considered the gold standard method for diagnosing common conditions of the lower urinary tract such detrusor overactivity (DO) and bladder outlet obstruction (BOO). However, with increasing concern about their "invasiveness" and associated potential patient morbidity, there has been a search towards non-invasive techniques such as ultrasound, computed tomography (CT), PET, magnetic resonance imaging (MRI), with the potential of becoming the mainstay diagnostic tools for LUTD. Furthermore, clinical assessment of the urethral symptoms is challenging and often requires further evaluation with imaging.

3.1 Ultrasonography

Ultrasonography (US) has over the years emerged as the most widely used imaging technique for the study of the LUT. In the past, US was identified as a technique of approach and guidance for the evaluation of LUT, but it is now recognized worldwide as the investigation of choice allowing precise diagnosis of many pathological conditions of the LUT, usually obviating the need for further radiological examinations. For instance, Transabdominal US is a cheap and easy modality to evaluate structural abnormalities of the bladder, stone disease of the bladder, post-void residual urine (PVR) or vesico-ureteral junction, neoplasms and inflammatory disorders [20].

The US, although simple to use, safe and acceptable by majority of patients, still remains real-time operator dependent, and in the light of new applications, requires experienced and skilled operator in whose hands often becomes the only exam needed to be able to direct the next phase of the diagnostic algorithm. Recent advances in US, incorporating a high resolution multi frequency transducers allows a meticulous study of the kidneys, its size, location and parenchymal structure, including a thorough assessment of the urinary bladder, perivesical space as well as pelvicalyceal and ureteral dilatation [21]. The use of US requires when possible a full bladder which is not distended to the extent that the individual has pain. This is necessary because, it is only a well-distended bladder that allows true mass abnormalities to be seen, or else, apparent focal wall diverticula or masses can be stimulated by invaginations of the deflated bladder, usually obscuring true bladder lesions such as calculi by the non-distended bladder folds [22].

In the assessment of LUT using US, patients are normally examined in the supine position but sometimes is required when there is the need to differentiate mobile intravesical abnormalities such as foreign bodies or stones from fixed lesions. The use of a 3.5–5-MHz curved array is normally acceptable for most US examinations of the LUT, however, with regards to anterior bladder wall, higher frequency linear probes are sometimes required for better resolution [22].

3.1.1 Ultrasonographic methods in the assessment of LUTD

Ultrasonography has proven to be essential in the evaluation of patients with lower urinary tract dysfunction (LUTD). This is based on the premise that LUTD may result in an alteration of the anatomic structures of the lower urinary tract (LUT) and vice versa [23]. In routine practice, US is mostly used to accurately measure the post-void residual urine (PVR) which indicates how completely an individual empties his bladder. Individuals with bladder outlet obstruction (BOO) and/or detrusor underactivity are commonly associated with elevated PVR [24]. The ultrasound measurement of bladder wall thickness (BWT) has also been linked to the diagnosis of overactive bladder (OAB) and BOO, with several studies reporting that increases in BWT can be a valuable biomarker for detrusor overactivity (DO) in subjects with an OAB syndrome [25, 26]. This is based on the assumption that increased BWT in BOO or OAB is secondary to hypertrophy of the detrusor wall, which is associated with increased isometric detrusor contraction against a competent urethral sphincter. These contractions lead to a rise in intravesical pressure, giving the individual a very strong desire to void [27]. Furthermore, it is generally accepted that an increase in mean BWT is unique to DO, with a study recording a statistically significant correlation between DO and BWT [27]. Detrusor wall thickness (DWT) might be a more accurate measure for BOO. A DWT >2 mm has been reported in 94% of men with signs of BOO on urodynamics [28]. In addition, measurement of DWT or BWT with US can used to examine the response to surgical or medical treatment of BOO. For instance, reduced BWT is detected after treatment with α-1 receptor blockers and transvesical prostatectomy [29, 30]. The ultrasonographic sections of the urinary bladder are defined from outside-in as bladder hyperechoic (adventitia), hypoechoic (detrusor muscle) and hyperechoic (bladder mucosa) [31, 32]. DWT measures only the middle layer, while the measurement of BWT involves all the three layers. The only issue with BWT measurement is that, it is volume dependent, and bladder wall thickness decrease with increasing filling volume. Hence, there is the need to measure bladder weight which should remain constant at different bladder volumes. Thus, with the aid of US, bladder weight is calculated from the thickness of the bladder wall and the intravesical volume assuming a spherical bladder (see **Figure 1**).

The benefit of utilizing US to monitor the deformation in the detrusor muscle have been shown by a recent study [33]. This provides insight into the detrusor muscle's dynamic and structural properties related to bladder pressure. In the study, it was demonstrated that US could be used to estimate strain in the detrusor muscle, which was positively correlated with the detrusor pressure. This suggests a possibility of using US in a real time manner to monitor detrusor muscle activity. Also, this

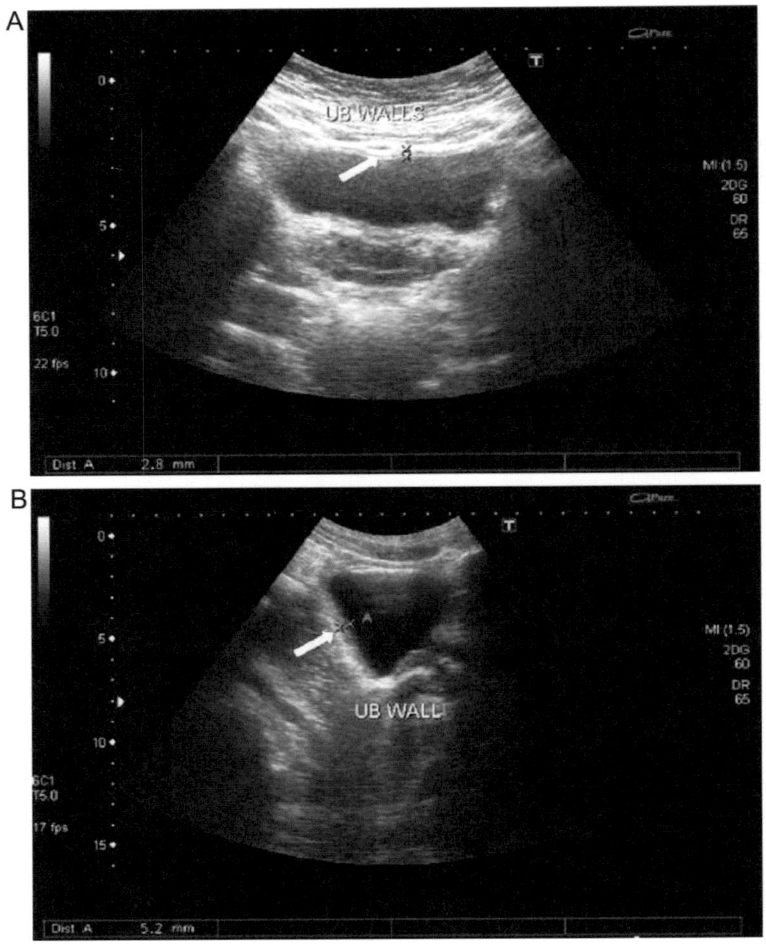

Figure 1.
(A) An ultrasound image of the urinary bladder (transverse scan) showing normal bladder wall thickness (BWT) (a, arrow) in a middle-aged woman with irritative lower urinary tract symptoms (LUTS) and normal filling cystometry (FCM); (B) ultrasound image (longitudinal scan) showing increased BWT (b, arrow) in a middle-aged man with irritative LUTS and detrusor overactivity [26].

finding is important because, it is an indication that US imaging could be used as a non-invasive modality option to replace the pressure flow studies which remain the standard diagnostic urodynamic tests for lower urinary tract symptoms (LUTS).

With recent advances in US imaging of the urethra, imaging of different structural abnormalities such as urethral neoplasms and urethral diverticulae are now possible. The typical symptoms of urethral diverticula are dyspareunia, urethral pain and post-voiding dribbling [34]. In addition, the multiplanar US allows imaging of the size, location, content, and configuration of the diverticulum. Also, in the case of surgical planning, US allows the diverticulum neck can to be evaluated, together with the presence of calculi in sac [20].

3.1.2 Recent innovations in the field of ultrasonography

The recent years have seen an evolution in the field of ultrasonography, with the introduction of applications which have great importance in the assessment of LUT. These new applications include harmonic imaging, motion-mode, transperineal US and 3D and 4D ultrasound.

Harmonic imaging (HI) is based on the harmonic response generated by the tissue or, when used by the contrast medium, rather than on the reflection of the fundamental frequency of the ultrasound beam. This provides a better definition of the profiles, particularly of the fluid structure systems, such as reduces artifacts; improves the representation of the contrast medium; and dilated collectors. Thus, HI removes low frequency sonic artifact which is usually the result of reverberation artifact and help better define the bladder wall. Motion-mode (M-mode) assists in the assessment of movement, and is therefore valuable in providing documentation and semiquantitative evaluation of ureteral peristalsis. Transperineal US, incorporating high-frequency linear probes allows ideal visualization of the vagina, urethra and surrounding structures. 3D and 4D US offer a multiaxial illustration of the entire kidney and bladder, thus improving renal parenchymal volume calculation, mostly in hydronephrosis or irregularly shaped kidneys. This is possible because, the dilated collecting system can be deducted from the overall kidney volume. Also, the potential of creating rendered views will allow the comprehensive demonstration of complex pathology [21, 35].

3.2 Voiding cystourethrogram X-ray (VCUG) of LUTD

VCUG uses a small amount of radiation to make images of an individual's urinary system, and it enables the assessment of the bladder's size and shape and also looks for abnormalities, such as a blockage along the path of the urine [36]. Images from VCUG can also show whether the urine is moving in the right direction. The normal flow of urine is from the kidneys down to the bladder through the ureters. However, in a condition called vesicoureteral (VU) reflux, urine flows backward from the bladder to one or both ureters and sometimes to the kidneys, and it sometimes occurs only at the voiding stage [37]. VU reflux can be detected by VCUG, which also includes taking X-ray images while the bladder is being emptied. This makes VCUG appropriate for diagnosing VU that only occurs while voiding [38].

During VCUG, a patient's bladder is filled with contrast material, followed by an X-ray machine used to send beams of radiation through the abdomen and pelvis, and images are recorded on special film or a computer. These images help physicians see problems in parts of the urinary system, including the bladder, urethra (the tube connecting the bladder with the outside of the body), and the ureters (the tubes connecting the kidneys to the bladder) (LUT), aiding in diagnosing LUTDS [39].

3.3 Magnetic resonance imaging in the assessment of LUTD

Technological advancement in imaging modalities, allowing cross-sectional imaging of the LUT is essential for further functional and/or morphological evaluation. Primary disorders for MRI of the LUT are bladder tumors and congenital abnormalities, and in addition, MRI is usually employed as a secondary imaging modality, particularly for assessing voiding dysfunction in pediatric urology [40]. MRI can also be used in conjunction with US for imaging of the size, content and position of the urethral diverticulae (see **Figure 2**). With regards to urethral neoplasms, MRI can reveal different characteristics of the different types of the neoplasms (see **Figure 2**). These neoplasms of the urethra appear as more heterogeneous lobulated, deeply infiltrating or exophytic lesions [20]. Urethral hypermobility can also be identified on both MR imaging and US, and it has been linked with stress urinary incontinence in women [42].

Currently, MRI is the only imaging modality that provides outstanding functional imaging and anatomical information without the use of ionizing radiation.

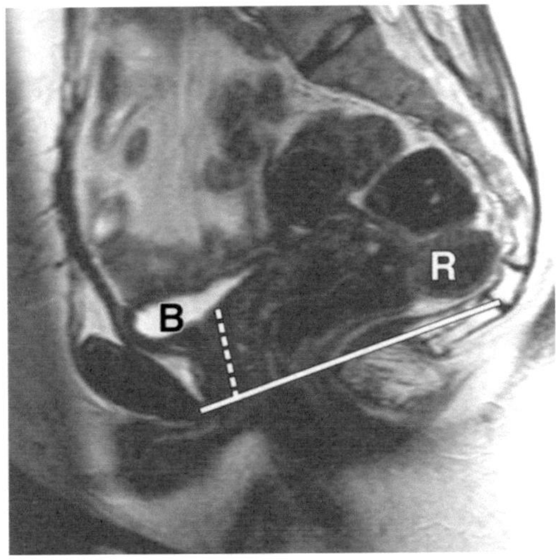

Figure 2.
A woman undergoing MRI evaluation of possible urethral diverticulum. Patient had previously undergone hysterectomy. Midline sagittal T2-weighted TSE image (6000/116, flip angle, 180°) obtained at rest shows no significant prolapse. Solid line represents pubococcygeal line, above which all pelvic organs are located. B = bladder, dotted line = urethra, R = rectum. Adapted from Bennett et al. [41].

MR imaging, in the light of rapid technological changes is now faster with less movement artifact, and therefore improved image quality and resolution. It allows an overall evaluation of the renal parenchyma, excretory cavity, surrounding tissue, together with the main vessels. The dynamic contrast enhancement of MRI is comparable to renal scintigraphy, and thus ensures a higher contrast spatial and temporal resolution. As a result of this inherently superior contrast resolution, MRI of the pelvis provides much better anatomical visualization than CT. Furthermore, heavy T2-weighted MRI is well suited for imaging of the urinary bladder, since the organ is filled with fluid, thus improving bladder visualization. With the advent of diffusion weighted MRI, in which imaging and MRI signals are weighted toward the diffusion characteristics of water, evaluation of LUT neoplasms, particularly bladder cancer has been done [21].

The evident advantages of MRI include the lack of both nephrotoxic contrast media and ionizing radiation required for CT, thus making it particularly suitable for imaging during renal failure and pregnancy. As a result, indications for MRI have been increasing rapidly over the years, and it is currently used as the standard imaging modality for staging pelvic cancers. In fact, it is better than CT for the anatomical depiction of the bladder wall [22].

3.4 Computed tomography in the assessment of LUTD

The combination of contrast studies and US scan have revolutionized imaging of LUT, pinpointing many of the clinical problems originating in the bladder. CT has become a vital complementary tool in the investigation of several disorders, and crucial for staging cancers. Thus, CT imaging is often employed in the staging of bladder cancer, however, its utility in the evaluation of LUTD remains limited. CT is the standard imaging modality for the study of adult urology, with or without contrast medium for the detection of stones [22]. Key advantages of CT are in providing detailed demonstration of overall bladder and pelvic anatomy.

Considering the fact that CT examination is highly radiant, its diagnostic potential cannot be transferred carelessly to children, since they have a higher radio sensitivity, smaller structures, lesser representation of adipose tissue, different tissue composition and different diseases, contrary to that of adults. Also, CT is not suitable for imaging of the urethra, penis and prostate, which are better assessed with MRI. That is, CT has limitations when applied to the urinary tract beyond the bladder.

Nevertheless, recent technological advancement in CT, incorporating multi-slice scanning with the possibility of isotropic imaging have further enhanced the precision of CT. In isotropic imaging, the block (or voxel) of imaging is acquired as a perfect cube, and is thus as dimensionally accurate as possible. Therefore, the 3D reconstruction of the contrast-filled bladder is rendered precisely, and virtual cystoscopy is possible. Thus, CT urography is being touted as one-stop imaging of the entire urinary tract, with the potential to replace conventional contrast studies and ultrasound, but this however requires further technical developments.

3.5 Positron emission tomography and functional MRI in the assessment of LUTD

Positron emission tomography (PET) and functional magnetic resonance imaging (fMRI) are powerful non-invasive tools utilized in the study of the supra-spinal control of the LUT directly through imaging of the brain. fMRI measures the changing proportion of deoxygenated and oxygenated hemoglobin in activated brain centers, while PET needs the injection of a radioactive isotope that will accumulate in a metabolically active brain region [20]. fMRI has a superb spatial and temporal resolution but needs multiple runs of the same event to increase signal-to-noise ratio, while PET is very sensitive for small changes in neural activity but not able to detect rapid changes in brain metabolism [42, 43].

Near infrared spectroscopy (NIRS) is occasionally utilized in the study of supraspinal control of the bladder. NIRS takes advantage of the varying concentrations of hemoglobin in the cerebral cortex, but its key disadvantage is the very limited resolution for deeper brain structures since it can only accurately measure to a depth of 1 cm beneath the skull [44].

In recent years, these different brain imaging techniques have been widely spread and optimized, providing a vast amount of literature about nearly every human cortical function. Unfortunately, the number of studies that have looked into brain control of bladder function is until now still relatively small, but nevertheless these studies have provided us with valuable new insights into LUT pathophysiology.

3.6 Imaging modalities as surrogates to urodynamic tests for the clinical assessment of BOO and DO

Lower urinary tract symptoms alone are usually not sufficient in diagnosing common complications of the LUT such as BOO, DO and BPE. Hence, in most cases, other investigations are required.

Uroflowmetry, though cheaper and easy to perform in clinical setting, is limited by its lack of specificity and inability to differentiate between BOO and detrusor underactivity. In much the same way, pressure-flow studies which serve as gold standard for diagnosing BOO are able to provide key information on the presence of obstruction as well as detrusor contractility. But this come at a cost, as urodynamic tests are invasive and require specialist equipment and training to perform tests and interpreted results, coupled with associated potential patient morbidity.

Therefore, the search for non-invasive diagnostic tests as potential replacement for these urodynamic tests, especially for the diagnosis of BOO, has been ongoing for many years. As such, parameters such as PVR, free uroflowmetry and quantification of prostate volume has been investigated. However, over the past two decades, the interest has been on BWT, DWT and bladder wall weight, owing to the rationale that BOO and DO are associated with an increase in bladder wall thickness and detrusor hypertrophy. These parameters (BWT, DWT) has been shown by several studies to be diagnostic of BOO and DO. Ultrasonography has thus emerged as the easiest and non-invasive option capable of measuring BWT, DWT and bladder wall weight, thus potentially obviating the need to resort to cumbersome and invasive urodynamic tests to diagnose BOO and DO (see **Figure 1**).

4. Conclusion

Imaging techniques can contribute prominently to our current understanding of lower urinary tract dysfunction. A variety of imaging modalities is available to visualize the urethra, bladder, prostate and pelvic floor. These techniques can be used to enhance our current knowledge of LUT pathophysiology and confirm clinical diagnosis, as an alternative diagnostic method to replace invasive urodynamic studies.

Acknowledgements

We acknowledge the entire staff of Spectra Health Imaging and Interventional Radiology for their valuable support during the preparation of this work.

Conflict of interest

The authors declare no conflict of interest.

Author details

George Asafu Adjaye Frimpong[1,2]*, Evans Aboagye[2,3] and Akosua Asafu-Adjaye Frimpong[2]

1 Department of Radiology, Kwame Nkrumah University of Science and Technology, Kumasi, Ghana

2 Spectra Health Imaging and Interventional Radiology, Kumasi, Ghana

3 Department of Molecular Medicine, Kwame Nkrumah University of Science and Technology, Kumasi, Ghana

*Address all correspondence to: george.frimpong@spectrahealthgh.com

References

[1] Morrison J, Birder L, Craggs M, De Groat WC, Downie J, Drake M, et al. Neural control. In: Abrams P, Cardozo L, Khoury S, Wein A, editors. Incontinence. Jersey: Health Publications, Ltd; 2005. pp. 363-422

[2] Fry CH, Brading AF, Hussain M, Lewis SA, Takeda M, Tuttle JB, et al. Cell biology. In: Abrams P, Cardozo L, Khoury S, Wein A, editors. Incontinence. Jersey: Health Publications, Ltd; 2005. pp. 313-362

[3] De Groat WC. Integrative control of the lower urinary tract: Preclinical perspective. British Journal of Pharmacology. 2006;**147**(S2):S25-S40. DOI: 10.1038/sj.bjp.0706604

[4] De Groat WC, Yoshimura N. Pharmacology of the lower urinary tract. Annual Review of Pharmacology and Toxicology. 2001;**41**(1):691-721

[5] National Clinical Guideline Centre. Urinary incontinence in neurological disease: Management of lower urinary tract dysfunction in neurological disease

[6] Panicker JN, Fowler CJ, Kessler TM. Lower urinary tract dysfunction in the neurological patient: Clinical assessment and management. The Lancet Neurology. 2015;**14**(7):720-732. DOI: 10.1016/S1474-4422(15)00070-8

[7] Patel AK, Chapple CR. Anatomy of the lower urinary tract. Surgery (Oxford). 2008;**26**(4):127-132. DOI: https://doi.org/10.1016/j.mpsur.2008.03.011

[8] Klingler HC, Madersbacher S, Djavan B, Schatzl G, Marberger M, Schmidbauer CP. Morbidity of the evaluation of the lower urinary tract with transurethral multichannel pressure-flow studies. The Journal of Urology. 1998;**159**(1):191-194. DOI: 10.1016/S0022-5347(01)64054-0

[9] De Groat WC. Anatomy and physiology of the lower urinary tract. The Urologic Clinics of North America. 1993;**20**(3):383

[10] Coyne KS, Sexton CC, Vats V, Thompson C, Kopp ZS, Milsom I. National community prevalence of overactive bladder in the United States stratified by sex and age. Urology. 2011;**77**(5):1081-1087. DOI: 10.1016/j.urology.2010.08.039

[11] Dorph S. Imaging of the lower urinary tract. In: Chest, Musculoskeleton, GI and Abdomen, Urinary Tract. Milano: Springer; 1996. pp. 154-158

[12] Wein AJ. Classification of neurogenic voiding dysfunction. The Journal of Urology. 1981;**125**(5):605-609. DOI: 10.1016/S0022-5347(17)55134-4

[13] Abrams P, Cardozo L, Fall M, Griffiths D, Rosier P, Ulmsten U, et al. The standardisation of terminology of lower urinary tract function: Report from the Standardisation Sub-committee of the International Continence Society. Neurourology and Urodynamics. 2002;**21**(2):167-178. DOI: 10.1002/nau.10052

[14] Sexton CC, Coyne KS, Kopp ZS, Irwin DE, Milsom I, Aiyer LP, et al. The overlap of storage, voiding and postmicturition symptoms and implications for treatment seeking in the USA, UK and Sweden: EpiLUTS. BJU International. 2009;**103**:12-23. DOI: 10.1111/j.1464-410X.2009.08369.x

[15] Wein AJ, Andersson KE, Drake MJ, Dmochowski RR. Bladder Dysfunction in the Adult: The Basis for Clinical Management. New York: Springer; 2014. DOI: 10. 1007/978-1-4939-0853-0

[16] Goldman HB, Zimmern PE. The treatment of female bladder outlet

obstruction. BJU International. 2006;**98**(2):359-366. DOI: 10.1111/j.1464-410X.2006.06335.x

[17] Ke QS, Kuo HC. The promise of bladder wall thickness as a useful biomarker for objective diagnosis of lower urinary tract dysfunction. Tzu Chi Medical Journal. 2011;**23**(1):1-8. DOI: 10.1016/j.tcmj.2011.03.005

[18] Abrams P, Cardozo L, Fall M, Griffiths D, Rosier P, Ulmsten U, et al. The standardisation of terminology in lower urinary tract function: Report from the Standardisation Sub-committee of the International Continence Society. Urology. 2003;**61**(1, 1):37-49. DOI: 10.1016/S0090-4295(02)02243-4

[19] Hashim H, Abrams P. Is the bladder a reliable witness for predicting detrusor overactivity? The Journal of Urology. 2006;**175**(1):191-194. DOI: 10.1016/S0022-5347(05)00067-4

[20] Deruyver Y, Hakim L, Franken J, De Ridder D. The use of imaging techniques in understanding lower urinary tract (dys) function. Autonomic Neuroscience. 2016;**200**:11-20. DOI: 10.1016/j.autneu.2016.05.008

[21] Taghizadeh A. Pediatric urology. In: Lima M, Manzoni G, editors. Contemporary Strategies from Fetal Life to Adolescence. Mailand: Springer-Verlag; 2015. DOI: 10.1007/978-88-470-5693-0

[22] Patel U, Rickards D. Imaging and Urodynamics of the Lower Urinary Tract. London: Springer; 2010. DOI: 10.1007/978-1-84882-836-0

[23] Yang JM, Huang WC. Bladder wall thickness on ultrasonographic cystourethrography. Journal of Ultrasound in Medicine. 2003;**22**(8):777-782. DOI: 10.7863/jum.2003.22.8.777

[24] Abrams PH, Griffiths DJ. The assessment of prostatic obstruction from urodynamic measurements and from residual urine. British Journal of Urology. 1979;**51**(2):129-134. DOI: /10.1111/j.1464-410X.1979.tb02846.x

[25] Khullar V, Cardozo LD, Salvatore S, Hill S. Ultrasound: A noninvasive screening test for detrusor instability. BJOG : An International Journal of Obstetrics and Gynaecology. 1996;**103**(9):904-908. DOI: 10.1111/j.1471-0528.1996.tb09910.x

[26] Cruz F, Heesakkers J, Khullar V, Tubaro A. Bladder wall thickness in overactive bladder: Does it have a role? European Urology Supplements. 2009;**8**(9):769-771. DOI: 10.1016/j.eursup.2009.05.002

[27] Ali MM, Ahmed AF, Khaled SM, Abozeid H, AbdelMagid ME. Accuracy of ultrasound-measured bladder wall thickness for the diagnosis of detrusor overactivity. The African Journal of Urology. 2015;**21**(1):25-29. DOI: 10.1016/j.afju.2014.11.005

[28] Oelke M, Höfner K, Jonas U, Ubbink D, de la Rosette J, Wijkstra H. Ultrasound measurement of detrusor wall thickness in healthy adults. Neurourology and Urodynamics: Official Journal of the International Continence Society. 2006;**25**(4):308-317. DOI: 10.1002/nau.20242

[29] Tubaro A, Carter S, Hind A, Vicentini C, Miano L. A prospective study of the safety and efficacy of suprapubic transvesical prostatectomy in patients with benign prostatic hyperplasia. The Journal of Urology. 2001;**166**(1):172-176. DOI: 10.1016/S0022-5347(05)66102-2

[30] Egilmez T, Pourbagher MA, Guvel S, Kilinc F, Turunc T, Ozkardes H. Effects of selective alpha-1-adrenergic receptor blockers on bladder weight. Urologia Internationalis. 2006;**76**(1):42-50. DOI: 10.1159/000089734

[31] Jequier S, Rousseau O. Sonographic measurements of the normal bladder wall in children. American Journal of Roentgenology. 1987;**149**(3):563-566. DOI: 10.2214/ajr.149.3.563

[32] Kojima M, Inui E, Ochiai A, Naya Y, Ukimura O, Watanabe H. Ultrasonic estimation of bladder weight as a measure of bladder hypertrophy in men with infravesical obstruction: A preliminary report. Urology. 1996;**47**(6):942-947. DOI: 10.1016/S0090-4295(96)00059-3

[33] Idzenga T, Farag F, Heesakkers J, Feitz W, de Korte CL. Noninvasive 2-dimensional monitoring of strain in the detrusor muscle in patients with lower urinary tract symptoms using ultrasound strain imaging. The Journal of Urology. 2013;**189**(4):1402-1408. DOI: 10.1016/j.juro.2012.09.165

[34] Romanzi LJ, Groutz A, Blaivas JG. Urethral diverticulum in women: Diverse presentations resulting in diagnostic delay and mismanagement. The Journal of Urology. 2000;**164**(2):428-433. DOI: 10.1016/S0022-5347(05)67377-6

[35] Riccabona M. Pediatric three-dimensional ultrasound: Basics and potential clinical value. Clinical Imaging. 2005;**29**(1):1-5. DOI: 10.1016/j.clinimag.2004.08.003

[36] Ključevšek D, Battelino N, Tomažič M, Kersnik Levart T. A comparison of echo-enhanced voiding urosonography with X-ray voiding cystourethrography in the first year of life. Acta Paediatrica. 2012;**101**(5):e235-e239. DOI: 10.1111/j.1651-2227.2011.02588.x

[37] Kenda RB. Imaging techniques for the detection of vesicoureteric reflux: What and when? Nephrology, Dialysis, Transplantation. 2001;**16**(1):4-7. DOI: 10.1093/ndt/16.1.4

[38] Nakamura M, Shinozaki T, Taniguchi N, Koibuchi H, Momoi M, Itoh K. Simultaneous voiding cystourethrography and voiding urosonography reveals utility of sonographic diagnosis of vesicoureteral reflux in children. Acta Paediatrica. 2003;**92**(12):1422-1426. DOI: 10.1111/j.1651-2227.2003.tb00826.x

[39] Darge K, Higgins M, Hwang TJ, Delgado J, Shukla A, Bellah R. Magnetic resonance and computed tomography in pediatric urology: An imaging overview for current and future daily practice. Radiologic Clinics. 2013;**51**(4):583-598. DOI: 10.1016/j.rcl.2013.03.004

[40] Macura KJ, Genadry RR, Bluemke DA. MR imaging of the female urethra and supporting ligaments in assessment of urinary incontinence: Spectrum of abnormalities. Radiographics. 2006;**26**:1135-1149

[41] Bennett GL, Hecht EM, Tanpitukpongse TP, Babb JS, Taouli B, Wong S, et al. MRI of the urethra in women with lower urinary tract symptoms: Spectrum of findings at static and dynamic imaging. American Journal of Roentgenology. 2009;**193**(6):1708-1715. DOI: 10.2214/AJR.08.1547

[42] Catana C, Drzezga A, Heiss WD, Rosen BR. PET/MRI for neurologic applications. Journal of Nuclear Medicine. 2012;**53**(12):1916-1925. DOI: 10.2967/jnumed.112.105346

[43] Mier W, Mier D. Advantages in functional imaging of the brain. Frontiers in Human Neuroscience. 2015;**9**:249. DOI: 10.3389/fnhum.2015.00249

[44] Matsumoto S, Ishikawa A, Matsumoto S, Homma Y. Brain response provoked by different bladder volumes: A near infrared spectroscopy study. Neurourology and Urodynamics. 2011;**30**(4):529-535. DOI: 10.1002/nau.21016

Chapter 4

Stress Urinary Incontinence: A Proteomics Overview

Goran Mitulović, Thomas Mohr and Marianne Koch

Abstract

Proteomics research offers one strategy to elucidate the etiology of stress urinary incontinence (SUI) by identification of a significant and sufficient number of proteins, which provides the ability to avoid a preselection of candidate proteins for a possible early detection of the SUI. SUI represents both a psychological as well as an economic burden, and prevalence rates are expected to increase in the future, due to increasing of life expectancy. The classical epidemiology of SUI is well understood, with many environmental and lifestyle risk factors identified, including age, obesity, parity, vaginal delivery, and family history. Despite this, much of the etiology of SUI remains unclear, and it is difficult to predict which women are at risk. This chapter shows some results based on proteomic analysis of the urine proteome, which might give the answer to the question on pathways activated in SUI. Besides proteins originating from the blood, urine contains proteins secreted from the inner wall of the bladder and the urethra, and these proteins might explain the processes involved in genesis of SUI.

Keywords: stress urinary incontinence, urinary proteome, proteomics

1. Introduction

Stress urinary incontinence (SUI) is a disorder observed with the female population with widely varying prevalence, which is estimated to be 15–80%. The condition represents both a psychological and an economic burden, and it is expected that prevalence rates shall increase in the future, mainly due to increasing of life expectancy.

While the classical epidemiology of SUI is understood quite well, many environmental and lifestyle risk factors leading to the condition have been identified. Among others, these are age, obesity, parity, vaginal delivery, and family history of SUI. Despite this much of the etiology of SUI remains unclear, and it is difficult to predict which women are at risk.

Proteomic research offers one strategy to elucidate the etiology of SUI by identification of a significant and sufficient number of proteins, which provides the ability to avoid a preselection of candidate proteins. Many different serum, urine, and/or tissue protein markers have been investigated in the context of SUI. Almost all studies have targeted specific proteins as putative biomarkers, but with typically negative results. Prior studies have investigated a role for serum C-reactive protein, serum relaxin, and serum estradiol, without finding significant associations with symptoms.

 IntechOpen

2. Materials and methods

2.1 Samples

In order to generate valid data and exclude possible false-positive and false-negative samples being analyzed, urinary and serum samples from patients affected by stress incontinence cases and a proven history of symptoms of SUI for at least 3 months were obtained. This included a specific history of complaint of involuntary leakage on effort or exertion or on sneezing or coughing, a positive provocation stress test, which was defined as an observed transurethral loss of urine simultaneous with a cough or Valsalva maneuver at a bladder volume of minimum 300 ml. Furthermore, negative urine dipstick testing was necessary; all patients were older than 18 years and capable of independent toileting and having at least one previous vaginal delivery. In accordance with rules of the Medical University of Vienna, written informed consent was obtained from all participants. We excluded patients who had previous treatment for SUI (either surgical or pharmacological), a history of overactive bladder symptoms, and/or urinary incontinence other than SUI (tested using the ICIQ-UI Short Form questionnaire) [1]. In addition, a history of neurological disorders potentially affecting the urinary tract system, such as multiple sclerosis, Parkinson's disease, pelvic organ prolapse stage ≥ II (International Continence Society classification), clinically significant bladder outlet obstruction, and/or post-void residual volume > 100 ml, was also exclusion criteria. A series of other criteria were also observed, as described in Koch et al. [2]: the history of acute urinary retention or history of repeated catheterizations; history of bladder cancer or previous operation on the urinary tract; acute or recurrent urinary tract infection and/or hematuria; history of urinary tract stones, renal insufficiency, and hepatic disease; history of alcohol and/or drug abuse; pregnancy or lactation; and finally any patient with a serious medical condition.

Participants in the control group met identical criteria, but with no symptomatic SUI (ICIQ-short form score equal to 0) and negative cough stress test. Urine samples were obtained once only without requirement for a specific time of day. Participants were given a sterile urine cup (maximum 50 ml) and asked to deliver the first-void urine. In addition we retrieved blood samples from peripheral veins of all participants to determine their creatinine, transaminase, and bilirubin status. Urine samples were stored in the refrigerator at 4°C for a maximum of 1 hour before they were taken to the Clinical Institute of Laboratory Medicine (Proteomics Core Facility) for immediate processing.

2.2 Proteomics sample preparation

Trypsin for protein digestion was purchased from Promega Inc. (Vienna, Austria). Solvents for high-performance liquid chromatography (HPLC)—methanol (MeOH), acetonitrile (AcN), 2,2,2-trifluoroethanol (TFE), formic acid (FA), heptafluorobutyric acid (HFBA), iodoacetamide (IAA), triethyl bicarbonate (TEAB), and dithiothreitol—were purchased from Sigma-Aldrich (Vienna, Austria).

Protein precipitation from urine was performed according to the internally modified Wessel-Fluege method for protein precipitation, and all solvents were kept at −20°C. All working steps were performed on ice and centrifugation in a cooled centrifuge at +4°C. A sample volume of 2 ml of each urine sample was mixed with 6 ml methanol and 2 ml dichloromethane in a 50 ml Falcon tube, and samples were vigorously vortexed. After adding 6 ml of water to each sample, solutions were vortexed another time. Samples were subsequently stored at −20°C for a minimum of 20 minutes for enhancement of protein precipitation. Phase separation was carried out by subsequent centrifugation for 5 minutes at 4500 rounds per minute (rpm). The upper layer of the solution was then carefully discarded while keeping the interphase and lower layer, and additional 6 ml of methanol were added prior to vigorous vortexing. Final centrifugation was performed for 5 minutes. The resulting supernatant was carefully removed, and the remaining protein pellet was dried on air. The dried protein pellet was later dissolved in 200 μl of 50 mM triethylammonium bicarbonate (TEAB) at pH 8.5. In cases where the protein pellet could not be properly dissolved in 200 μl of 50 mM TEAB, additional 50–1000 μl 50 mM TEAB were added, and the sample was sonicated by using the ultrasonic cell disruptor (Ultrasonic Cell Disruptor, Branson 5200, Dietzenbach, Germany).

Blood samples were prepared as described by Koch et al. [3]. Briefly, samples were immediately centrifuged to separate serum from blood cells and then frozen in separate vials at −20°C until further processing and an in-solution enzymatic digestion of all proteins extracted from both urinary and serum samples were achieved by applying a combination of Glu-C and trypsin (Promega, Vienna, Austria). This combination was selected in order to achieve improved sequence coverage for proteins. All steps for sample preparation were performed using previously published protocols [4–6].

2.3 Chromatographic separation and detection

Peptide separation was achieved using nano-high-performance liquid chromatography on a nano-RSLC Ultimate 3000 system (ThermoFisher Scientific, Vienna, Austria) using the PepMap C18 column (75 μm ID × 50 cm length, 3 μm ID, 100 Å pore size, ThermoFisher Scientific, Vienna, Austria). The separation column was mounted in a column oven and operated at 60°C. Prior to the separation on the nano-separation column, peptides were loaded onto a trap column (300 μm ID × 5 mm length, PepMap 300 Å pore size, ThermoFisher Scientific, Vienna, Austria). The analysis of biological samples bears the risk of carry-over and contamination of subsequent runs in cases where injected samples contained high amounts of peptides. Therefore, separation system was flushed between sample injections using the method developed earlier and described by Mitulovic et al. [7]. Optimization of loading conditions have been described in a number of other publications; however, we have used the conditions described in a paper by Schöbinger et al. where loading mobile phase was cooled to 3°C in order to enable improved peptide trapping on the trap column, which was operated at 60°C.

Details on separation gradient formation and mobile phases used are described in publications by Koch et al. [2, 3].

Mass spectrometric detection of digested peptides was performed using the maXis Impact time-of-flight (qToF) MS (Bruker, Bremen, Germany) equipped with the Captive Spray nano-electrospray source and operated at 1.6 kV; source temperature was set to 180°C for effective desolvatization of the analytes introduced from LC. Peptide masses were scanned in the range of m/z 300–m/z 2000, and 20 most intense signals were selected for MS/MS fragmentation. Fragmentation was performed by using collision-induced dissociation with nitrogen in the CID cell. Single-charged ions were excluded from MS/MS fragmentation, and those carrying charges of +2 to +4 were fragmented. In order to ensure fragmentation of a maximum number of ions, already fragmented masses were excluded from further fragmentation for 60 seconds but were allowed if the following MS/MS intensity was three times higher as compared to the previous MS/MS peak intensity. All measurements were performed in triplicate to provide corrections for technical variability of chromatographic separation and the ionization.

2.4 Data analysis

In order to identify proteins in analyzed sample, database search of mass spectrometric data was performed using the Human Swiss-Prot Database in its actual version at the time of analysis. Details of data search are described by Koch et al. [3]. Briefly, all searches were performed using Mascot v. 2.51 (http://www.matrixscience.com/). For the database search, trypsin and Glu-C were selected as enzymes with carbamidomethyl on Cys as fixed modification and oxidation on Met, phosphorylation on Ser, Thr, and Tyr as variable modifications.

Protein abundance was estimated by using peptide counts normalized to counts per million (cpm). Log2-fold change was estimated based on variance stabilized average log2 cpm values using the package edgeR. Resulting p values were corrected for multiple testing according to Burden et al. [8].

3. Results

Only proteins identified with at least two detected and identified peptides were selected for further analysis.

3.1 Proteins identified in urinary samples

The total number of identified individual proteins in the case group was 1459 and 2148 in the control group. The median number of identified proteins per urine sample was 377 (range 1167) in the case group and 417 (range 1197) in the control group.

Only 6 of the 828 proteins showed a significant difference in abundance in urine samples. This difference between SUI and controls was observed with a q-value <0.25. Out of these six identifications, three known proteins showed a higher abundance in SUI samples compared to controls: plasma serine protease inhibitor (logFC 1.11), leucine-rich alpha-2-glycoprotein (logFC 3.91), and lysosomal alpha-glucosidase (logFC 1.24). From three uncharacterized proteins, one protein (gene symbol: PPIA) also showed higher abundance in SUI samples (logFC 1.96), whereas the other two uncharacterized proteins (gene symbol, UMOD; gene symbol, KIAA0586) presented a lower abundance in SUI samples than controls (logFC-4.87; logFC-1.99, respectively). **Table 1** shows the proteins identified in urinary samples with significant difference between the control and the case group.

Protein	Gene symbol	LogFC	q-value
Plasma serine protease inhibitor	SERPINA5	1.111	0.029
Leucine-rich alpha-2-glycoprotein	LRG1	3.909	0.019
Lysosomal alpha-glycosidase	GAA	1.237	0.062
Uromodulin	UMOD	−4.867	0.002
Peptidyl-prolyl cis-trans isomerase A	PPIA	1.962	0.227
TALPID3 (KIAA0586)	TALPID3 (KIAA0586)	−1.992	0.227

Table 1.
Proteins identified with a significantly different abundance in urine of patients with stress urinary incontinence (SUI) compared to control samples.

4. Discussion

Current study is not the first one describing the urinary proteome [9–13]. However, this study was the first one to address specific clinical problem of SUI. The methodology used for both sample preparation and sample analysis was kept as simple as possible so that it can be easily reproduced in any proteomic laboratory without adaptations of existing hardware.

Figure 1 shows the typical chromatogram for separation of tryptic peptides from a patient's urinary sample. The large number of peaks in the chromatogram indicates the presence of a large number of peptides. Database search revealed that in almost all cases of urinary proteomic analysis, the major proteins being identified are serum albumin and uromodulin. This is physiologically normal and common, although a common knowledge implies that no proteins or, at least, very low number of proteins shall be present in the urine.

4.1 Proteins identified

Uromodulin, being the major urinary protein, was a major hit following serum albumin.

The study identified six different, putative, probably SUI-specific urinary proteins for the first time.

The abundance of all these proteins was found to be higher in SUI samples, and these are plasma serine protease inhibitor (SERPINA5), leucine-rich alpha-2-glycoprotein (LRG1), and lysosomal alpha-glucosidase (GAA).

The results showing the enrichment of mentioned proteins based on KEGG pathway analysis are shown in **Figure 2**.

SERPINA5 is usually present in urine in very low concentrations and serves, among other functions, as a pro-inflammatory factor, which might be an explanation for it overexpression in samples of patients with SUI [1, 14–20]. Furthermore, SERPINA5 was recently mentioned in a number of publications addressing diverse medical conditions, including pediatric leukemia, breast cancer, HIV infection, and hepatocellular carcinoma, which have identified a role played by SERPINA5 during disease development [21–24].

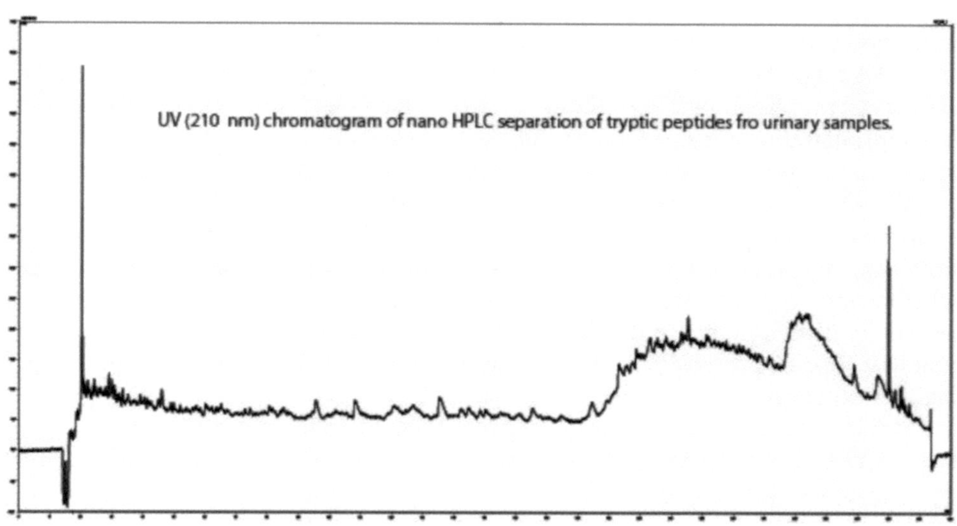

Figure 1.
UV Chromatogram trace at 210 nm showing the separation of tryptic peptides from urinary sample.

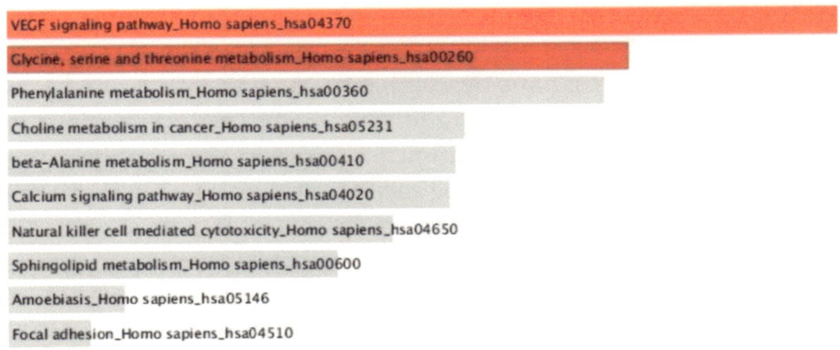

Figure 2.
KEGG pathway for the set of proteins with affected expression in SUI samples.

Another protein, the leucine-rich alpha-2-glycoprotein, was also found to be increased in samples of SUI patients. This protein is secreted and normally present in plasma; however, it was also described to be involved in nonspecific inflammatory and cancer processes [25–28]. It has recently been described in the context of ulcerative colitis activity, pediatric, invasive bladder cancer, biliary tract cancer, lung cancer, pancreatic cancer, heart failure, neutrophilic granulocyte differentiation, and autoimmune diseases [29, 30].

Lysosomal alpha-glucosidase, another protein with increased expression in SUI samples, is essential for the degradation of glycogen to glucose in lysosomes, and it is present in, basically, all cells. Mutations in the respective gene result in Pompe disease, a severe and devastating glycogen storage disease caused by a deficiency in acid α-glucosidase. This condition is characterized by the lack of lysosomal alpha-glucosidase, which leads to intralysosomal accumulation of glycogen, the final consequence of which is the failure of the heart and skeletal muscles. The Pompe disease is being treated by enzyme replacement therapy. However, this is not sufficient, although it helps preventing assisted patients' ventilation and ensuring a ventilation-free survival. GAA is an enzyme that is essential for lysosomal glycogen hydrolysis, and the protein has also been identified as a potential biomarker for gut wall integrity in infants with necrotizing enterocolitis, an inflammatory process involving the intestinal tissue [31]. GAA has not been described as a factor for SUI, but the involvement of GAA in pathologies of smooth muscle [32] suggests that this protein might have an important role for the proper function of the bladder. Niedworok et al. [33] suggested that GAA might be involved in bladder cancer as an endogenous inhibitor of bladder cancer cell proliferation. The authors concluded that GAA is upregulated in response to antiproliferative tyrosine kinase inhibitors. That would mean that high biglycan expression is associated with favorable prognosis for patients with bladder cancer.

Alsaikhan et al. [34] investigated the partial bladder obstruction and the expression, among other factors, of GAA. Authors describe that small leucine-rich proteoglycans, required for collagen fibrillogenesis showed a significant reduction, which was consistent with a pro-fibrotic environment and deregulated collagen assembly. Although this study did not address the matter of incontinence, it showed that leucine-rich proteoglycans have an important role to play for the regulation of bladder function.

A similar observation was made by Appunni et al. [35, 36] for the role of leucine-rich proteoglycans and the bladder cancer. Leucine-rich proteoglycans are not only required in the matrix for structural framework, but they also show to be effective in controlling various physiological functions. Among these functions are also the cell cycle regulation and the leucine-rich proteoglycans which perform the role of the guardians of the cellular matrix.

Upon database search and quantitation, peptidyl-prolyl cis-trans isomerase A (PPIA) was found to be overexpressed. This protein has been described to be involved in inflammatory processes and immunomodulation and induction of interleukin-6 release from macrophages. Recent publications have discussed an involvement in type 2 diabetes mellitus, vascular disease, and gastric adenocarcinoma [31].

Two of the identified uncharacterized proteins, which are encoded by associated with the genes UMOD and KIAA0586, showed lower expression in SUI samples.

UMOD encodes for the protein uromodulin, which is, among other functions, involved in the prevention of urinary tract infection, water/electrolyte balance, and kidney innate immunity. Uromodulin is usually highly abundant in the urine of healthy humans, and, as mentioned previously, it is the most abundant protein in normal urine [37]. Interestingly, uromodulin is another glycoprotein identified to have different expression patterns in SUI samples as compared to control samples. UMOD is a GPI-anchored glycoprotein produced by the kidney but not derived from the blood. The function of these proteins is still not well understood, but it is taught to be linked to the water/electrolyte balance and kidney innate immunity. Hypertension in pregnancy was associated with a decrease in the uromodulin's excretion rate [38], and the results of SUI samples also revealed that the level of uromodulin was decreased. Furthermore, UMOD can be used as a predictive factor for preeclampsia [39]. UMOD has been described to prevent the binding of the IgG light chain to their putative receptors [40]. Da Silva et al. described the role of UMOD as an allergen epitope [41] for activation of the allergy-associated T cells in mouse. There is no description of causality in humans; however, the lower expression of this protein in samples of SUI patients might be of importance considering the function of the smooth muscle of the urinary bladder.

KIAA0586 encodes for the protein TALPID3, which is required for ciliogenesis and sonic hedgehog/SHH signaling [42–48]. Fleming et al. [49] described the possible involvement of TALPID3 in kidney damage in patients with Joubert syndrome. Interestingly, all patients enrolled in this study and having a mutation on KIAA05866 gene, which encodes for TALPID3, showed to have significantly better chances of preserving the kidneys, which are, otherwise, affected by the Joubert syndrome. It is still unclear why this protein was identified with a decreased abundancy in samples of SUI patients.

Another protein that was ubiquitous in all samples was keratin. Keratin is commonly identified during proteomics analysis, and it often serves as a quality control of the analysis, if not present in high amounts. However, more often, keratin is considered being a contaminant and something that shall be kept out of the sample by any means.

Therefore, requirements were taken to exclude any possible contamination with keratin, but it was still identified in large amount in all samples. Besides being considered a contaminant for proteomics experiments, keratin is an important part of the urinary proteome which seems to be present in all collected samples.

As for now, no biomarkers have yet been identified for SUI, and it is rather improbable that a single protein will be a marker. A more probable scenario is that a group of proteins with a significantly different abundance in SUI patients compared to controls will be defined as putative markers.

The best chance to identify these proteins will be by investigating the known functions, tissue specificities, and interactions of the specific proteins identified in samples of SUI patients. It is also important to gain a detailed insight into potential mechanisms of the pathophysiology and etiology of SUI, which seem to depend on many factors and might be a complex process depending on more physiological processes taking place in the urinary bladder. Proteins, which were identified with significantly higher abundance in SUI samples, have been described earlier as active participants in inflammatory processes and cancer development. On the other hand, proteins that were identified and quantified with a significantly lower abundance usually seem to have a protective effect in the urinary tract system although we cannot be explained at the current time.

5. Conclusion

It is important to stress out that one of the most important factors for a successful analysis is the selection of samples to be analyzed. It is very important to include urine samples retrieved from a population with very strict inclusion and exclusion criteria in order to avoid confounding factors. Urine samples must be processed according to a standardized protocol within a short time frame after collection.

Although a thorough map of the human proteome has been described, and made available to researchers [50], this map is still not complete and it is prone to errors and biases. Therefore, the incomplete "humane proteome mapping" is an additional challenge despite efforts of the research community to identify and characterize all human proteins.

By investigating the urinary proteome at one time point only, no conclusion can be made on whether the significantly differently expressed proteins are a consequence of the pathological process or whether they themselves are directly involved in causal processes.

Therefore, due to the characteristics of the identified proteins, it can be said that inflammatory processes may be involved in the etiology of SUI. However, the relevance of these findings regarding the pathogenesis of SUI needs to be broadly investigated, and the results described need to be replicated in a different population and at different time points.

Author details

Goran Mitulović[1,2]*, Thomas Mohr[3] and Marianne Koch[4]

1 Clinical Department of Laboratory Medicine, Medical University of Vienna, Vienna, Austria

2 Proteomic Core Facility, Medical University of Vienna, Vienna, Austria

3 Science Consult Thomas Mohr KG, Guntramsdorf, Austria

4 Clinical Division of General, Gynecology and Gynecologic Oncology, Department of Obstetrics and Gynecology, Medical University of Vienna, Vienna, Austria

*Address all correspondence to: goran.mitulovic@meduniwien.ac.at

References

[1] Johannessen HH, Stafne SN, Falk RS, Stordahl A, Wibe A, Morkved S. Prevalence and predictors of double incontinence 1 year after first delivery. International Urogynecology Journal. 2018;**29**(10):1529-1535

[2] Koch M, Mitulovic G, Hanzal E, Umek W, Seyfert S, Mohr T, et al. Urinary proteomic pattern in female stress urinary incontinence: A pilot study. International Urogynecology Journal. Nov 2016;**27**(11):1729-1734

[3] Koch M, Umek W, Hanzal E, Mohr T, Seyfert S, Koelbl H, et al. Serum proteomic pattern in female stress urinary incontinence. Electrophoresis. 2018;**39**(8):1071-1078

[4] Fichtenbaum A, Schmid R, Mitulović G. Direct injection of HILIC fractions on the reversed-phase trap column improves protein identification rates for salivary proteins. Electrophoresis. 2016;**37**(22):2922-2929

[5] Schöbinger M, Klein OJ, Mitulović G. Low-temperature mobile phase for peptide trapping at elevated separation temperature prior to nano RP-HPLC–MS/MS. Separations. 2016;**3**:6

[6] Mitulovic G, Panic-Jankovic T, Pietrowski D, Gorshkov M, Schmid R. Analyzing the preimplantation secretome of human embryos. FEBS Journal. 2013;**280**:499-500

[7] Mitulović G, Stingl C, Steinmacher I, Hudecz O, Hutchins JRA, Peters J-M, et al. Preventing carryover of peptides and proteins in nano LC-MS separations. Analytical Chemistry. 2009;**81**(14):5955-5960

[8] Burden CJ, Qureshi SE, Wilson SR. Error estimates for the analysis of differential expression from RNA-seq count data. PeerJ. 2014;**2**:e576

[9] Aregger F, Uehlinger DE, Witowski J, Brunisholz RA, Hunziker P, Frey FJ, et al. Identification of IGFBP-7 by urinary proteomics as a novel prognostic marker in early acute kidney injury. Kidney International. 2014;**85**(4):909-919

[10] Court M, Selevsek N, Matondo M, Allory Y, Garin J, Masselon CD, et al. Toward a standardized urine proteome analysis methodology. Proteomics. 2011;**11**(6):1160-1171

[11] Marimuthu A, O'Meally R, Chaerkady R, Subbannayya Y, Nanjappa V, Kumar P, et al. A comprehensive map of the human urinary proteome. Journal of Proteome Research. 2011;**10**(6):2734-2743

[12] Nagaraj N, Mann M. Quantitative analysis of the intra- and inter-individual variability of the normal urinary proteome. Journal of Proteome Research. 2011;**10**(2):637-645

[13] Marimuthu A, O'Meally RN, Chaerkady R, Subbannayya Y, Nanjappa V, Kumar P, et al. A comprehensive map of the human urinary proteome. Journal of Proteome Research. 2011;**10**(6):2734-2743

[14] Colla C, Paiva LL, Ferla L, Trento MJB, de Vargas IMP, Dos Santos BA, et al. Pelvic floor dysfunction in the immediate puerperium, and 1 and 3 months after vaginal or cesarean delivery. International Journal of Gynaecology and Obstetrics. 2018;**143**(1):94-100

[15] Li YT, Lee WL. Is it really risky for postpartum stress urinary incontinence in the first year postpartum. Journal of the Chinese Medical Association: JCMA. 2018;**81**(6):582

[16] Daly D, Clarke M, Begley C. Urinary incontinence in nulliparous

women before and during pregnancy: Prevalence, incidence, type, and risk factors. International Urogynecology Journal. 2018;**29**(3):353-362

[17] Kokabi R, Yazdanpanah D. Effects of delivery mode and sociodemographic factors on postpartum stress urinary incontinency in primipara women: A prospective cohort study. Journal of the Chinese Medical Association: JCMA. 2017;**80**(8):498-502

[18] Volloyhaug I, van Gruting I, van Delft K, Sultan AH, Thakar R. Is bladder neck and urethral mobility associated with urinary incontinence and mode of delivery 4 years after childbirth? Neurourology and Urodynamics. 2017;**36**(5):1403-1410

[19] Martin-Martin S, Pascual-Fernandez A, Alvarez-Colomo C, Calvo-Gonzalez R, Munoz-Moreno M, Cortinas-Gonzalez JR. Urinary incontinence during pregnancy and postpartum. Associated risk factors and influence of pelvic floor exercises. Archivos espanoles de urologia. 2014;**67**(4):323-330

[20] Gartland D, Donath S, MacArthur C, Brown SJ. The onset, recurrence and associated obstetric risk factors for urinary incontinence in the first 18 months after a first birth: An Australian nulliparous cohort study. BJOG : An International Journal of Obstetrics and Gynaecology. 2012;**119**(11):1361-1369

[21] Kawahara R, Bollinger JG, Rivera C, Ribeiro AC, Brandao TB, Paes Leme AF, et al. A targeted proteomic strategy for the measurement of oral cancer candidate biomarkers in human saliva. Proteomics. 2016;**16**(1):159-173

[22] Priola GM, Foster MW, Deal AM, Richardson BM, Thompson JW, Blatt J. Cerebrospinal fluid proteomics in children during induction for acute lymphoblastic leukemia: A pilot study. Pediatric Blood & Cancer. 2015;**62**(7):1190-1194

[23] Jing Y, Jia D, Wong CM, Oi-Lin Ng I, Zhang Z, Liu L, et al. SERPINA5 inhibits tumor cell migration by modulating the fibronectin-integrin beta1 signaling pathway in hepatocellular carcinoma. Molecular Oncology. 2014;**8**(2):366-377

[24] Haynes BP, Viale G, Galimberti V, Rotmensz N, Gibelli B, Smith IE, et al. Differences in expression of proliferation-associated genes and RANKL across the menstrual cycle in estrogen receptor-positive primary breast cancer. Breast Cancer Research and Treatment. 2014;**148**(2):327-335

[25] Smith C, Batruch I, Bauca J, Kosanam H, Ridley J, Bernardini M, et al. Deciphering the peptidome of urine from ovarian cancer patients and healthy controls. Clinical Proteomics. 2014;**11**(1):23

[26] Tung CL, Lin ST, Chou HC, Chen YW, Lin HC, Tung CL, et al. Proteomics-based identification of plasma biomarkers in oral squamous cell carcinoma. Journal of Pharmaceutical and Biomedical Analysis. 2013;**75**:7-17

[27] Andersen J, Boylan K, Jemmerson R, Geller M, Misemer B, Harrington K, et al. Leucine-rich alpha-2-glycoprotein-1 is upregulated in sera and tumors of ovarian cancer patients. Journal of Ovarian Research. 2010;**3**:21

[28] Kay RG, Barton C, Velloso CP, Brown PR, Bartlett C, Blazevich AJ, et al. High-throughput ultra-high-performance liquid chromatography/tandem mass spectrometry quantitation of insulin-like growth factor-I and leucine-rich alpha-2-glycoprotein in serum as biomarkers of recombinant human growth hormone administration. Rapid Communications in Mass Spectrometry. 2009;**23**(19):3173-3182

[29] Serada S, Fujimoto M, Ogata A, Terabe F, Hirano T, Iijima H, et al. iTRAQ-based proteomic identification of leucine-rich alpha-2 glycoprotein as a novel inflammatory biomarker in autoimmune diseases. Annals of the Rheumatic Diseases. 2010;**69**(4):770-774

[30] Serada S, Fujimoto M, Terabe F, Iijima H, Shinzaki S, Matsuzaki S, et al. Serum leucine-rich alpha-2 glycoprotein is a disease activity biomarker in ulcerative colitis. Inflammatory Bowel Diseases. 2012;**18**(11):2169-2179

[31] Ramachandran S, Venugopal A, Kutty VR, A V GD, Chitrasree V, et al. Plasma level of cyclophilin A is increased in patients with type 2 diabetes mellitus and suggests presence of vascular disease. Cardiovascular Diabetology. 2014;**13**:38

[32] McCall AL, Salemi J, Bhanap P, Strickland LM, Elmallah MK. The impact of Pompe disease on smooth muscle: A review. Journal of Smooth Muscle Research. 2018;**54**:100-118

[33] Niedworok C, Röck K, Kretschmer I, Freudenberger T, Nagy N, Szarvas T, et al. Inhibitory role of the small leucine-rich proteoglycan biglycan in bladder cancer. PLoS One. 2013;**8**(11):e80084

[34] Alsaikhan B, Fahlman R, Ding J, Tredget E, Metcalfe PD. Proteomic profile of an acute partial bladder outlet obstruction. Canadian Urological Association Journal—Journal de l'Association des urologues du Canada. 2015;**9**(3-4):E114-EE21

[35] Appunni S, Anand V, Khandelwal M, Gupta N, Rubens M, Sharma A. Small Leucine Rich Proteoglycans (decorin, biglycan and lumican) in cancer. Clinica Chimica Acta. 2019;**491**:1-7

[36] Appunni S, Anand V, Khandelwal M, Seth A, Mathur S, Sharma A. Altered expression of small leucine-rich proteoglycans (Decorin, Biglycan and Lumican): Plausible diagnostic marker in urothelial carcinoma of bladder. Tumor Biology. 2017;**39**(5):1010428317699112

[37] Liu M, Chen Y, Liang Y, Liu Y, Wang S, Hou P, et al. Novel UMOD mutations in familial juvenile hyperuricemic nephropathy lead to abnormal uromodulin intracellular trafficking. Gene. 2013;**531**(2):363-369

[38] Nesselhut T, Rath W, Grunow E, Kaufholz G, Ostermai U, Cillien N, et al. The relationship between urinary Tamm-Horsfall glycoprotein excretion and urinary activity of glycosidases in normal pregnancy and pre-eclampsia. European Journal of Obstetrics, Gynecology, and Reproductive Biology. 1993;**48**(1):23-31

[39] Carty DM, Siwy J, Brennand JE, Zürbig P, Mullen W, Franke J, et al. Urinary proteomics for prediction of preeclampsia. Hypertension. 2011;**57**(3):561-569

[40] Franciscus Petrus Nijkamp AD-K, Redegeld FAM, De WJG. Joseph VanGestur Vidarsson Inventor. Means and Methods for Manipulating Hypersensitivity-Like Responses. Den Haag, The Netherlands: European Union; 2003

[41] da Silva Antunes R, Pham J, McMurtrey C, Hildebrand WH, Phillips E, Mallal S, et al. Urinary Peptides as a novel source of T cell allergen epitopes. Frontiers in Immunology. April 2018;**9**:886

[42] Wang L, Failler M, Fu W, Dynlacht BD. A distal centriolar protein network controls organelle maturation and asymmetry. Nature Communications. 2018;**9**(1):3938

[43] Ojeda Naharros I, Cristian FB, Zang J, Gesemann M, Ingham PW, Neuhauss SCF, et al. The ciliopathy protein TALPID3/KIAA0586 acts upstream

of Rab8 activation in zebrafish photoreceptor outer segment formation and maintenance. Scientific Reports. 2018;**8**(1):2211

[44] Wang L, Lee K, Malonis R, Sanchez I, Dynlacht BD. Tethering of an E3 ligase by PCM1 regulates the abundance of centrosomal KIAA0586/Talpid3 and promotes ciliogenesis. eLife. 2016;**5**

[45] Stephen LA, Tawamie H, Davis GM, Tebbe L, Nurnberg P, Nurnberg G, et al. TALPID3 controls centrosome and cell polarity and the human ortholog KIAA0586 is mutated in Joubert syndrome (JBTS23). eLife. 2015;**4**

[46] Malicdan MC, Vilboux T, Stephen J, Maglic D, Mian L, Konzman D, et al. Mutations in human homologue of chicken talpid3 gene (KIAA0586) cause a hybrid ciliopathy with overlapping features of Jeune and Joubert syndromes. Journal of Medical Genetics. 2015;**52**(12):830-839

[47] Alby C, Piquand K, Huber C, Megarbane A, Ichkou A, Legendre M, et al. Mutations in KIAA0586 cause lethal ciliopathies ranging from a hydrolethalus phenotype to short-rib polydactyly syndrome. American Journal of Human Genetics. 2015;**97**(2):311-318

[48] Bachmann-Gagescu R, Phelps IG, Dempsey JC, Sharma VA, Ishak GE, Boyle EA, et al. KIAA0586 is mutated in Joubert syndrome. Human Mutation. 2015;**36**(9):831-835

[49] Fleming LR, Doherty DA, Parisi MA, Glass IA, Bryant J, Fischer R, et al. Prospective evaluation of kidney disease in Joubert syndrome. Clinical Journal of the American Society of Nephrology: CJASN. 2017;**12**(12):1962-1973

[50] Kim M-S, Pinto SM, Getnet D, Nirujogi RS, Manda SS, Chaerkady R, et al. A draft map of the human proteome. Nature. 2014;**509**(7502):575-581

Section 3

Management

Chapter 5

Advances in Treatment of Nocturnal Enuresis in Children

Bingying Zhou, Jianxin Lu, Peiqi Shi and Yifang An

Abstract

Nocturnal enuresis is a condition with complex etiology affecting plenty of children and families. Even though multifarious clinical trials and studies have been designed and completed, some inconclusive results on nocturnal enuresis confuse clinicians. This article aims to provide useful information for clinicians by summarizing the existing evidence on nocturnal enuresis and discussing the effectiveness and safety of different treatments. Nocturnal enuresis mainly results from the disorders related to central nervous system, which may cause nocturnal polyuria, nighttime bladder capacity decline, arousal disorder, and various accompanying diseases. We discussed the efficacy and safety of different treatments for monosymptomatic nocturnal enuresis, including standard therapies, simple behavioral interventions, complex behavioral interventions, alarm therapy, desmopressin and other drugs, biofeedback therapy, electrical stimulation, acupuncture, Chinese herbal medicine, massage, and so on. Alarm is still the most effective single therapy with lower relapse rate. Desmopressin has efficacy mainly in children with nocturnal polyuria. Children with detrusor overactivity or decreasing functional bladder capacity can choose anticholinergics. Additionally, tricyclic drugs, biofeedback therapy, electrical stimulation, acupuncture, massage, and so on are therapeutic options for children with nocturnal enuresis.

Keywords: nocturnal enuresis, alarm, desmopressin, behavioral interventions, acupuncture

1. Introduction

Nocturnal enuresis (NE) is a common disease that pediatricians often encounter. It is defined as an intermittent involuntary micturition during sleep in children over 5 years of age with at least two episodes per week and duration of more than 3 months [1]. Basically, NE is divided into non-monosymptomatic nocturnal enuresis (NMNE) and monosymptomatic nocturnal enuresis (MNE) according to whether there are daytime lower urinary tract symptoms. On the other hand, it is also classified into primary nocturnal enuresis (PNE) and secondary nocturnal enuresis (SNE) according to whether or not the duration of dry days is less than 6 months [1]. Secondary NE requires clinicians to identify and evaluate the diseases which NE is secondary to and treat them first. In PNE, NMNE usually means that children have more complex bladder dysfunction or other potential pathology and need to be referred to a specialist for further diagnosis and treatment. Although some children with MNE can be self-healing and the prevalence gradually decrease with age [2], most treatments for NE cannot achieve high cure rates and may cause high relapse rates. This may result from the complexity and uncertainty of the etiology of NE and the use of inappropriate treatment.

2. Epidemiology

According to Jain et al.'s review, the prevalence of MNE varies from 3.8 to 18.9% in different countries [2]. The risk factors related to NE reported in different studies include constipation, positive family history, obstructive respiratory disorder, deep sleep, corporal punishment at school, urinary tract infection, etc. [3–6]. However, the effect of each factor on NE varies from study to study, and no universal conclusion is drawn. The results from different studies may be contradictory. For example, a few researches reported that the prevalence of NE was significantly higher in boys than the one in girls [3, 7], while other studies draw the opposite conclusion that girls' prevalence is higher [8]. The potential reasons for the contradiction of results in different studies performed in different countries may be related to the difference in diagnostic criteria followed by each survey, sample size, sampling method, questionnaire design, and cultural background in different regions. According to Wen's survey about NE in Chinese children, the overall prevalence was 4.07%, which is much lower than counterparts in other countries [9]. In it, Dr. Wen reported that Chinese parents would wake their children to void once they found children's dysphoria due to the fullness of the bladder. Besides, he also found that Chinese parents were more likely to withdraw the diaper for their children as early as possible, which is believed to be helpful for the children to build normal urination habits. Similar to the mechanism of alarm therapy, these actions may have a positive effect to promote the establishment of reflex between bladder filling feeling and urination. It is important to analyze epidemiological data, which may help us to understand the importance of the children and their parents' behavior and other complex physiological, pathological, and social psychological elements involved in the prevalence of NE.

3. Clinical diagnosis and treatment algorithm

There are a few diagnosis and treatment algorithms of NE proposed by the International Children's Continence Society (ICCS), the International Continence Society (ICS), and some other literatures with similarities and differences. In this part, the algorithm of the ICCS's practical consensus guideline is introduced and modified.

NE has many possible causes: genetic factors, renal physiological factors, deficiency of antidiuretic hormone (ADH, vasopressin) leading to nocturnal polyuria, bladder dysfunction, arousal disorder, maturation delay, circadian rhythm disorder, etc. Moreover, many associated diseases such as obstructive sleep-disordered breathing, constipation, fecal incontinence, attention deficit disorder (ADD) and attention deficit hyperactivity disorder (ADHD), obesity, psychological problems, etc. can also be seen in children with NE. These associated diseases should be identified in the clinical evaluation and be treated first. For children without those conditions, the increase in nocturnal urine production and nighttime bladder capacity reduction are the two main prototypes. To provide an outline in the diagnosis and management of NE, we build an algorithm after summarizing available guidelines. **Figure 1** is the clinical diagnosis and treatment algorithm adapted from the guideline of Walle et al [10]:

1. Clinical management tool is a medical history and symptoms collection form (see [10]).

2. Voiding diary (bladder diary) is not necessary.

3. After MNE is diagnosed, the 2012 guideline recommends directly the alarm and desmopressin treatment options. John Michael's review in 2014 recommends 6 weeks of urotherapy first and then evaluating the child to decide whether to take alarm or desmopressin [11].

4. EBC: expected bladder capacity, calculated as {30 + (age in years × 30)} in milliliters.

5. MVV: maximum voided volume, the largest urine volume of 24 h (see part bladder diary for details).

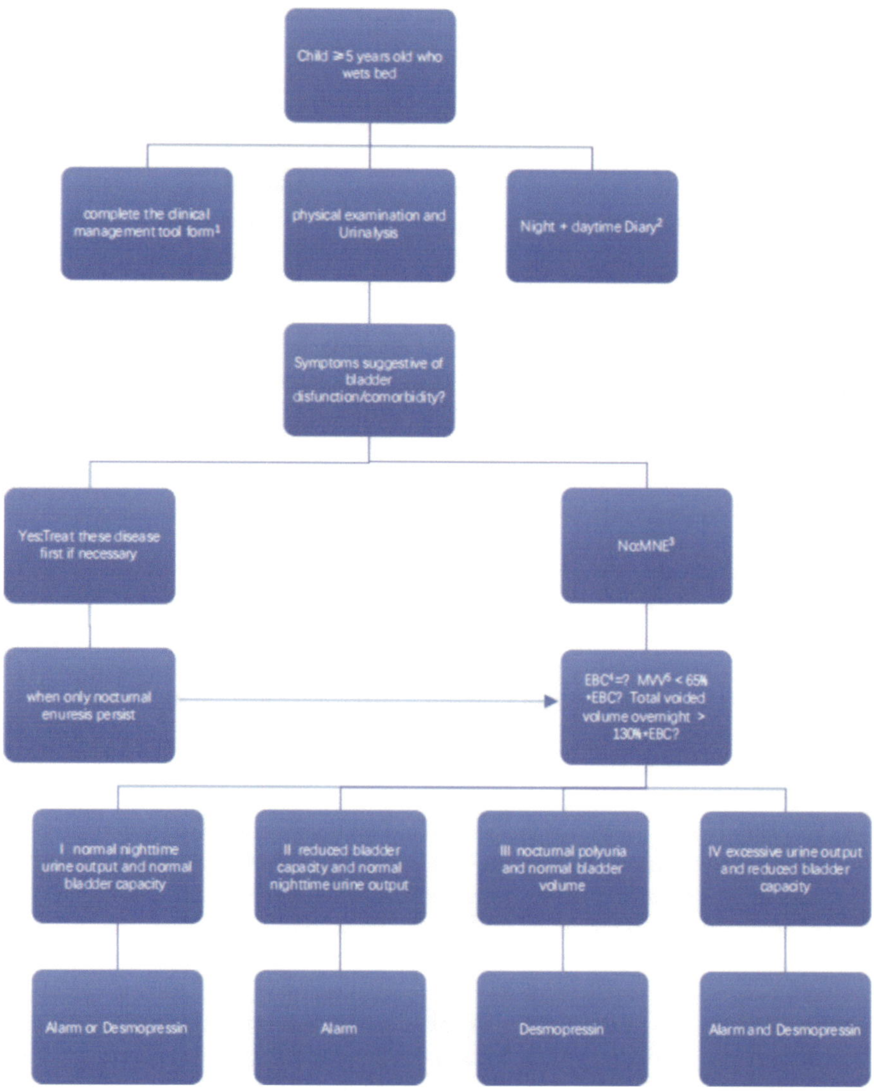
Child ≥5 years old who wets bed
complete the clinical management tool form1
physical examination and Urinalysis
Night + daytime Diary2
Symptoms suggestive of bladder disfunction/comorbidity?
Yes:Treat these disease first if necessary
No:MNE3
when only nocturnal enuresis persist
EBC4=? MVV5 < 65% *EBC? Total voided volume overnight > 130%*EBC?
I normal nighttime urine output and normal bladder capacity
II reduced bladder capacity and normal nighttime urine output
III nocturnal polyuria and normal bladder volume
IV excessive urine output and reduced bladder capacity
Alarm or Desmopressin
Alarm
Desmopressin
Alarm and Desmopressin

Figure 1.
Nocturnal enuresis algorithm (modified from Walle, 2012).

4. Treatment

4.1 Urotherapy

According to the 2006 ICCS's standardized terminology of lower urinary tract (LUT) function, urotherapy is defined as a nonsurgical and nonpharmacological treatment for LUT dysfunction [1]. It includes standard therapy which means the therapy is noninterventional and has specific interventions.

4.1.1 Standard therapy

The standard therapy usually has these components as below:

1. Health education. Health education refers to providing parents basic information about normal LUT function and the causes, risk factors, different treatments, and their implementation of MNE [1]. The clinicians should emphasize that the condition is common and can be healed by itself and that parents should have a positive attitude instead of thinking enuresis as a shame because this helps children to establish their motivation for active participation and reduce damage to their self-esteem, which is the key to treatment [12].

2. Lifestyle advice. Develop healthy drinking and eating habits: avoid foods or beverages that have a diuretic effect, such as theophylline or caffeine; eat early in the evening, with less oil and less salt; and no more water or food and fruit rich in fluid at least 2 h before going to bed. These all avoid excessive nighttime fluids in body which may lead to overmuch urine production during the night. However, for children with MNE, fluid restriction may have a risk of reducing bladder capacity resulting in a decrease in the ratio of bladder capacity to nocturnal urine output, and so nocturnal enuresis increases [13]. Therefore, adequate fluid intake during the day is important, especially during the morning and early afternoon hours [14]. It is also good for cultivating the child's feeling of bladder fullness. Moreover, a research indicates that holding exercises can increase the maximum voided volume of children with MNE, so it is better not to be active after dinner [15].

3. Developing regular voiding and bowel habits. As the ICCS recommended, children should develop a good habit of regular urination during the day and schedule to urinate before going to bed and in the early morning after waking up. The daily routine of micturition should be comprised of once in the morning, at least twice during school hours, and once each after school, at dinner, and before going to bed, with totally less than seven urinations during daytime [14]. Besides, parents should instruct the child to use a comfortable voiding posture to relax the pelvic floor muscles—and that means sitting on the toilet safely with the bottom and feet supported. Constipation is a common concomitant disease in children with NE, especially with NMNE. It is recommended to eat more foods rich in dietary fiber and develop regular bowel movements every day, best after breakfast. Based on current evidence, medication can be used to soften children's stools if necessary [14].

4. Voiding diary or bladder diary (VD or BD). According to the 2012 ICCS's practical consensus guidelines for MNE's management [10], BD is recommended to assess the children's voiding habit, especially for the families in which parents are unclear about children's voiding history. The most important function of BD is to evaluate the bladder capacity of children through daytime diary and

to assess the presence of nocturnal polyuria (NP) through nighttime diary. It is also helpful to distinguish NMNE through finding out daytime polyuria, stress urinary incontinence, urgency urinary incontinence, etc. *A daytime diary* should include at least fluid intake time, urination time, fluid intake volume, urination volume, and the occurrence of urinary incontinence and exclude the first urination after getting up in the morning. The recording time should be at least 3–4 consecutive days. Children attending school can choose to record two consecutive weekends [10]. In daytime diary, the most important thing that requires clinicians' attention is the largest urinated volume which can indicate the child's bladder capacity. It can be determined if the bladder capacity is reduced or increased when the maximum voided volume is <65% or >130% expected bladder capacity (EBC's calculation formula is shown in **Figure 1**). *The nighttime diary* should include at least urination time (if the child gets up to the toilet), urination volume, diaper weight overnight, first urination volume after getting up in the morning, dry night or not (there is any enuresis or not), and whether there is bowel movement that day. The recording time should be at least seven consecutive nights [10]. What the nighttime diary can tell the clinicians is the child's amount of urine produced at night by adding first urination after getting up in the morning, the nighttime diaper weight, and nocturnal urination volume to the toilet. If the total nighttime urine output exceeds 130% EBC, it is determined as nighttime polyuria (NP). Through analyzing individual BD, children with MNE can be classified into one of the four subtypes as shown in **Figure 1**. Then the corresponding treatment could be determined. In addition, by calculating a child's body surface area, we can find whether the 24-h urine volume >2 L/m^2, which means the child has polyuria; by observing a child's water taking, we can know if the child has polydipsia which is considered as a predictor of diabetes or kidney disease. It is worth noting that children with these conditions are not suitable to take desmopressin.

4.1.2 Specific interventions

Specific interventions comprise behavioral modification and nonbehavioral strategies including pelvic muscle floor training, biofeedback, electrical stimulation, etc. [1]. And the behavioral interventions can also be divided into simple and complex strategies based on whether it is a single action or they are composite interventions [16] (**Table 1**).

Simple behavioral Interventions	Reward systems
	Lifting or waking the children at night to urinate[1]
	Bladder training[2]
	Fluid restriction
	Cleanliness training
Complex behavioral interventions	Dry bed training (DBT)
	Full-spectrum home training (FSHT)
	Arousal therapy

[1]Lifting and waking therapy includes lifting with or without password and waking randomly or to a certain time.
[2]Bladder training includes retention control training, pelvic floor muscle training, sphincter control exercises, and stream interruption exercises.

Table 1.
Categories of behavioral interventions.

4.1.2.1 Simple behavioral interventions

Most of the simple behavioral interventions were initially presented in some early literatures, because the effects of first-line treatment on NE had not yet been determined at the time. They are often used in clinical treatment, but the efficacy is controversial since it lacks high-quality evidence. A systematic review about the efficacy and safety of simple behavioral interventions for NE has been published in the Cochrane Library. Unfortunately, only limited evidence is available. For most interventions only a single clinical trial was included, and therefore the data cannot be combined for meta-analysis except for the comparison between bladder training and alarm [16]. Furthermore, some other important limitations about the clinical trials were discussed in this review: for children with NE included in the trials, MNE and NMNE were not further distinguished; most trials had methodological deficiencies, and more than half of the trials reporting continuous outcomes did not report SDs; the trials' sample size was small, risk of bias was high, and the confidence interval was too wide; since there is a lack of long-term follow-up after the end of treatment, no data were available to assess the long-term efficacy of the interventions [16]. The following is a summary of this review's conclusion which needs to be cautiously referenced.

In the simple behavioral interventions referring to reward systems, lifting or waking the children, bladder training, and fluid restriction (*cleanliness training was not reviewed*), though all of them were more effective statistically than the control group, none of them had a better effect than others at the end of the treatment. When compared with alarm or different drugs, they were usually less effective except for bladder training which has no significant difference with drugs [16]. In terms of safety, adverse events were not reported in the included trials.

Bladder training is a behavioral therapy aiming to increase bladder capacity and strengthen the control of bladder in children. According to the review, bladder training seemed to be superior to the nonactive movements group in gaining less mean wet nights at the end of the treatment. However, there was no difference in the number of children who did not achieve 14 dry nights [16]. Another prospective trial further revealed that the basic bladder training's effects mostly were pronounced after the third month of treatment for the MNE children who did not receive any previous treatment. Therefore, for children who are not strongly willing to accept behavioral interventions, early administration of alarm or desmopressin is necessary [17]. But it seems to have good efficacy in children with NMNE [18].

Lifting without password is a controversial intervention because it allows the children to urinate while asleep, but it is useless to reduce the occurrence of nocturnal enuresis [19]. Being consistent with the conclusions of this review, a study also showed that the lifting without password group had a significantly higher proportion in the number of dry children than the control group and was even superior to lifting with password group and rewards group. In terms of long-term effect, both lifting groups had more dry children than the two other groups during 3 years follow-up [20].

4.1.2.2 Complex behavioral interventions

Dry bed training (DBT) is the oldest complex behavioral interventions with a multicomponent package of nighttime waking schedule, cleanliness training, reinforcement techniques, and other interventions. It has different versions and a few adapted versions with some components removed [21]. Full-spectrum home training (FSHT) is a combination with alarm, cleanliness training, and retention control training in the daytime. To maximize the effect, the FSHT needs to be overlearned (giving extra fluids at bedtime after successfully becoming dry). Specific implementation steps of DBT and FSHT have been described by Brown and Glazener [22, 23]. In a Cochrane review of NE, complex behavioral interventions were compared with control, alarm, and other complex behavioral interventions. Moreover, complex behavioral interventions removing alarm were compared with control, alarm, and complex behavioral interventions supplemented by alarm. The conclusions were that DBT or FSHT was better than control in efficacy and relapse rate and marginally superior to alarm alone. Either complex behavioral interventions removing alarm or control intervention was inferior to alarm alone or complex behavioral interventions supplemented by alarm. There is no evidence for the comparison between complex behavioral interventions removing alarm and control. Additionally, adverse events were not described by the trials [23]. Unfortunately, the included studies in the systematic review have some limitations including small scale, small quantity, and poor quality. Besides, it has to be mentioned that the interventions are heavy burdens on families.

Alarm and reward system are the components of arousal therapy/training, which was reported to have a high efficacy and low relapse rate in an early literature [24]. However, they have not been recommended by the guideline [10] because there is not enough clinical evidence, which is similar to FSHT [25].

4.1.2.3 Nonbehavioral interventions

Biofeedback therapy and electrical stimulation therapy were originally used to treat voiding dysfunction, and now they have been tried to treat refractory MNE or PNE with a reported good efficacy. Dr. Hoekx and his colleagues prospectively evaluated the effect of bladder biofeedback in 21 boys and 3 girls (mean age 10.4 years). After treatment 17/24 patients showed good response that means they achieved totally dry. During the 60-month follow-up, 4 patients were lost, 15 were dry at night, and 4 continued bed-wetting. The proportion of children with small bladder capacity in responders is much less than the one in non-responders [26]. In a randomized clinical trial published in 2015, 54 children with PNE were included and randomly divided into interferential (IF) electrical stimulation group and control group. A responding rate was reported as 55.5 and 22% in the IF and control group at the 1-year follow-up ($P = 0.01$), respectively. In terms of the mean number of dry nights per week and the mean improvement score, the IF group was superior compared to control group. Additionally, no adverse events were reported [27]. In another trial, children with refractory MNE were randomly assigned to intra-anal biofeedback with behavioral therapy, electrical stimulation with behavioral therapy, and pelvic floor muscle training groups. The trial stated a total efficacy of three groups in the outcomes and that intra-anal ES group was superior to BF training group. But in these three outcomes, the method to assess nighttime bladder capacity with morning first urine volume is not accurate [28]. In short, there is no adequate clinical evidence to determine the therapeutic effectiveness of these NE treatments (**Table 2**).

Nonbehavioral interventions	Biofeedback (BF)[1]
	Electrical stimulation (ES)

[1]*Including bladder biofeedback and intra-anal biofeedback*

Table 2.
Categories of nonbehavioral interventions.

4.2 Alarm

Alarm therapy, also known as enuretic alarm devices (EADs) or enuresis alarm treatment (EA), is a kind of therapy with sufficient evidence which shows a higher response rate and a superior long-time success than the control or other therapies. Although its relapse rate is still a little high, the addition of overlearning and dry bed training or avoiding penalties can reduce the rate by nearly half [29]. In terms of different types of alarms, there was no enough evidence to draw conclusions, neither did the comparison between alarm and other behavioral therapies [29]. Two other Cochrane reviews revealed that alarm had better effects than simple behavioral interventions, but not when compared with complex behavioral therapies [16, 23]. Some researchers believed the effect of alarm might be weakened if only the parents were waked by the alarm instead of the children. A result from Tsuji's study showed whether the parents or children themselves are waked by the alarm or the effectiveness of alarm is equal [30]. Apos E. et al.'s study published in 2018 stated excellent effects of alarm therapy for MNE, NMNE, PNE, and SNE children using alarm therapy and especially for NMNE children [31]. The ICCS guideline also recommended that the alarm should be considered as the therapeutic option for every child. Furthermore, those children who have motivated parents should be given a priority [14].

It has to be mentioned that alarm does not have an immediate effect. Normally, it often needs to take a period of time to achieve the expected efficacy. The appropriate course recommended by the ICCS is 2–3 months until children achieve 14 consecutive dry nights or the effect is not good [14]. Similarly, the ICS's recommendation is to evaluate the efficacy of alarm after at least 6–8 weeks [12]. It also states that the efficacy will increase with treatment duration; however, the ideal course of alarm has not been introduced [12]. In one study, a total of 455 children with PMNE were randomly divided into three groups and received 3, 4, and 5 months of uninterrupted alarm treatment, respectively. The results showed that children with 16–20 weeks' treatment had better curative effect [32]. Unfortunately, this study did not observe the effect with a longer follow-up. So we cannot conclude if the longer treatment can further increase the effect of alarm. In another study, NE children who were ineffective after 3 months' alarm treatment were randomized into two groups to receive a repeat alarm treatment for ≥3 months without interval and with an interval of more than 6 months, separately. The success rate in the latter group was significantly higher than the former, which means repeat alarm therapy with at least one interval may reawaken children's response [33]. Despite the small sample size, this study may provide new ideas for children who have no response to alarm treatment.

The possible mechanism of alarm therapy may be a gradual establishment of a conditioned reflex between bladder filling and waking. Evidence showed that it could increase the prepulse inhibition (PPI), similar to the effect of desamino-arginine vasopressin (dDAVP), which suggested that the alarm could also promote the maturation of the reflex control of NE [34]. In addition, a study reported that children's daytime functional bladder capacity increased markedly after treatment with alarm [35]. Therefore, the efficacy of alarm on children with NE may be achieved through multiple effects.

4.3 Desmopressin

Desmopressin is an arginine vasopressin analog that enhances the reabsorption of water by the distal convoluted tubules and collecting ducts of the kidney and inhibits the secretion of aldosterone. Schulz-Juergensen et al.'s study published in 2007 showed that 1-desamino-8-D-arginine vasopressin (dDAVP) could make

PMNE children's PPI upregulate to the age-related normal level. The authors offered a different explanation about dDAVP that it not only had a role in the kidney but also acted as a central neurotransmitter which has a positive effect on the delayed maturation of NE children's micturition reflex [36]. According to the results of this study, desmopressin has the ability to cure a substantial group of children with NE in theory. However, it is more complicated in practice with problems of how to choose the potential suitable children for desmopressin therapy. Moreover, what is the appropriate dose and course of treatment are also big issues. To assess the effect of desmopressin, a number of studies have been performed. Evidence showed that it could significantly reduce bed-wetting by 1–2 nights per week during the treatment, but there is no difference in wet nights per week compared with the placebo group. Additionally, when comparing with alarm therapy, lower effectiveness and higher subsequent relapse rate were reported in the desmopressin group according to a Cochrane review [37].

In general, children with nocturnal polyuria are suitable for desmopressin therapy. Basically, we can identify this subtype of MNE using the bladder diary. However, there is an evidence showing that children with NE may not present continuous nocturnal polyuria. Nocturnal urine production increases significantly on wet nights than the dry nights. Children without abnormal increase in nocturnal urine production do not respond to desmopressin [38]. This study revealed the polyuria characteristics for a subgroup of NE children and confirmed the efficacy of desmopressin for these children. Furthermore, some other studies also showed that desmopressin was not effective in children with low functional bladder capacity [39] and those with abnormal bladder volume and wall thickness (BVWT) [40], indicating that desmopressin's clinical use should carefully identify children with potential bladder dysfunction.

Referring to appropriate dose of desmopressin, there is an insufficient evidence to determine whether higher dose is more effective or not [37]. The recommended safe dose is 0.2–0.4 mg for tablets and 120–240 μg for melt formulation [14]. There is no enough evidence to state what is the appropriate course of treatment. Because of high relapse rate after treatment, it is advised to gradually reduce the drug dose instead of stopping it directly at the time of getting a complete response. For long-term safety, desmopressin is proven to be safe enough to use for several years. Water intoxication with hyponatremia is only a severe adverse event that needs to be concerned. Fluid restriction of 200 ml or less for the whole night is advised with desmopressin treatment [14]. Moreover, nasal spray reports more hyponatremia than oral formulations [41].

4.4 Pharmacotherapy (other than desmopressin)

Anticholinergic drugs are widely used for the management of NE since they can bind to choline receptors and produce antagonistic activity against acetylcholine and consequently relieve detrusor overactivity. They can be classified into M and N receptor blockers according to their selectivity for different receptors. M receptor blockers, also called as antimuscarinics, are more commonly used to treat NE. Generally, M receptors consist of five different subtypes, including M1, M2, M3, M4, and M5. Of those, M2 and M3 subtypes are mainly distributed in the bladder wall, and M3 has an upregulated expression in patients with overactive bladder. Therefore, the therapeutic mechanism of antimuscarinics is to inhibit the bladder M receptor, relax the detrusor, and consequently expand the bladder capacity. The mechanism determines that antimuscarinic drugs should be mainly used in treatment of NE children who are suffering from latent bladder smooth muscle spasm, detrusor overactivity, or decreased functional bladder capacity.

This kind of children usually has daytime symptoms of lower urinary tract and is classified as NMNE. However, some children diagnosed as MNE are also suitable for anticholinergic drug therapy because they have only nighttime detrusor overactivity or mild urinary tract symptoms during daytime. For children who do not respond to alarm or desmopressin therapy, anticholinergic agents are usually a kind of therapeutic option. The clinical application of anticholinergic drugs should focus on how to identify the children with indications through bladder diary and other diagnostic techniques. Studies to evaluate the efficacy of anticholinergic drugs and their combination with alarm or desmopressin on these children should be conducted as well.

Differing from anticholinergic drugs, the mechanism of tricyclic drugs in the treatment of NE is still unclear. The possible mechanism includes inhibiting rapid eye movement sleep to promote sleep arousal and stimulating antidiuretic hormone secretion. A Cochrane review showed that tricyclic drugs could reduce about one wet night per week, but most children relapsed after treatment which is similar to desmopressin and inferior to alarm [42]. In addition, most tricyclic drugs may cause serious side effects such as cardiotoxicity, so they are only used for the treatment of refractory or therapy-resistant NE. An exception is reboxetine. Neveus and his colleagues attempted to treat children with therapy-resistant NE using reboxetine, and they found that 59% of the patients reached a full response after 4 weeks of treatment. Moreover, during treatment, no significant cardiac toxicity was reported [43]. Lundmark et al. used reboxetine to treat therapy-resistant NE children and also achieved good results without significant cardiac adverse events [44]. Therefore, reboxetine may be a good therapeutic option instead of imipramine, but its effectiveness and safety need more clinical studies to prove.

4.5 Complementary and alternative approaches

Although a large amount of evidence has shown the effectiveness of conventional treatment including alarm and pharmacotherapy on NE [31, 45], these approaches cannot meet all the needs of the children and their parents. It is reported that as high as 30% of families discontinue the treatment of alarm on their own reason [46]. On the other hand, the side effects related to medications bother both children and their family members. Therefore, a number of parents are more likely to seek help from complementary and alternative medicine for their children. Being outside of conventional medicine, complementary and alternative medicine includes a series of medical approaches, such as acupuncture, herbal therapy, and massage. Recently, an increasing evidence has shown the efficacy of complementary and alternative medicine on management of NE.

4.5.1 Acupuncture

Acupuncture, as a component of traditional Chinese medicine, has been used to manage a number of chronic diseases. Even though acupuncture originates in China, its efficacy on various urological diseases has been recognized in industrial world [47]. A number of studies have demonstrated the effectiveness of acupuncture in treatment of NE. In a single-arm trial, Bjorkstrom et al. [48] showed that an 8-week treatment with 20 sessions of acupuncture decreased the episodes of NE and the sleep arousal threshold significantly in 65 and 50% of children, respectively, at the follow-up of 6 months. Another study further revealed that acupuncture might increase the nocturnal bladder capacity significantly in responders [49]. To assess the effect of acupuncture on NE, several systematic reviews were conducted. As presented in a part of Cochrane systematic review [50], Glazener et al. showed that acupuncture might result in a more significant improvement for children with NE than sham intervention. Moreover, acupuncture seemed to have a lower failure rate than combination therapy with meclofenoxate, oryzanol, and thiamine. Six years later, the updated Cochrane systematic review [50] demonstrated the same result. Another systematic review showed that acupuncture in conjunction with other treatment could reduce the number of NE more significantly than other treatment alone [51]. It needs to be mentioned that some methodological limitations have to be taken into consideration when we analyze the evidence. These systematic reviews included the nonrandomized and quasi-randomized studies besides randomized controlled trials, which may weaken the level of evidence. To provide the high quality of evidence, a recent published systematic review excluded nonrandomized and quasi-randomized trials and showed that acupuncture might be more effective in management of NE than sham procedure or drug treatment [52]. However, some studies with the intervention of acupoint injection were included in the systematic review, which may make the results controversial. As is known, acupuncture only provides physical effect, while both physical and chemical effects are involved in acupoint injection.

To further provide evidence, we designed and conducted a systematic review. After performing a comprehensive search of medical literature, including Cochrane Central Register of Controlled Trials, MEDLINE, EMBASE, CBM, ClinicalTrials.gov, and the World Health Organization International Clinical Trials Registry Platform, on February 22, 2019, a total of 238 randomized controlled trials were reviewed, and 10 of them with 953 randomized participants (441 in acupuncture group and 412 in control group) were included. We found that compared with the other treatment, acupuncture resulted in significantly higher complete response rate [OR = 2.41, 95%CI (1.41, 4.93) P = 0.002], so did the significance when compared with conventional drug, sham procedure, and herbal therapy, respectively. Moreover, although acupuncture did not reduce the average number of NE in comparison with other treatment, a significant decrease was found when compared to the sham intervention [MD = −1.49, 95%CI (−2.26, −0.72) P = 0.0002]. In terms of adverse events, there was no significant difference between acupuncture and other treatment [OR = 0.62, 95%CI (0.04, 8.72) P = 0.72]. Based on our results, acupuncture may have a better effect in management of NE, when compared to conventional drug, sham procedure, and herbal therapy, respectively.

The potential mechanism of acupuncture's effectiveness in managing NE might be the regulation on bladder function and secretion of antidiuretic hormone. A study assessed the effect of acupuncture on urodynamic parameters in children with NE and found acupuncture could suppress the detrusor overactivity [53]. On the other hand, an animal experiment showed that acupuncture could downregulate the concentration of arginine vasopressin in the hypothalamic paraventricular nucleus and upregulate the concentration of arginine vasopressin in the hypothalamic supraoptic nucleus, periaqueductal gray, caudate nucleus, and nucleus raphe magnus [54], which may cause an antidiuretic effect.

4.5.2 Herbal therapy

Herbal therapy is an important component of traditional medicine. About 3500 years ago, Papyrus Ebers described that cypress, juniper berries, and beer might be used to treat NE, which is the earliest record for the treatment of NE. Although there is lack of enough evidence, some herbs, such as St John's wort (*Hypericum perforatum*), infusions of horsetail, or corn silk (*Zea mays*), are considered to be helpful to regulate bladder function [55]. Hosein et al. performed a double-blind randomized controlled trial to evaluate the effectiveness of chamomile oil in treating NE, in which 80 patients were allocated to receive chamomile oil or placebo. After 2 weeks treatment, the patients' mean wet night frequency in chamomile oil group decreased from 8.2 to 5.6 nights/2 weeks, while no significant difference was found in placebo group [56]. We hope more clinical trials can provide more evidence for the efficacy of herbal therapy in future.

4.5.3 Massage and chiropractic

Both massage and chiropractic are a kind of manipulative therapy acting on the body with appropriate pressure. The former focuses on the relaxation of muscle, while the latter centers on the regulation of spinal articulations. They can be the therapeutic options for NE since their effectiveness has been reported. An early study attempted to treat five children with NE using massage which pressed the acupoint located in the creases between the first and the second and the third phalanx of the 5th finger. After an average of 20 sessions of therapy, two children achieved complete recovery, and one got partial recovery [57]. In another study, Yuksek et al. performed an efficacy comparison of massage with oxybutynin. After 6 months treatment, 83.3% of patients in massage group experienced a significant improvement, which is better than 58.3% in oxybutynin group [58].

In a case series study, 171 children with NE were treated by chiropractic. After 2 weeks treatment, the median episodes of NE decreased from 7.0 per week at baseline to 5.6 per week and further dropped to 4.0 per week at the end of treatment [59]. Another finding of the study is that the more severe symptoms children had, the less benefit they got from the treatment, which means those with mild to moderate NE might be suitable for chiropractic. Reed et al. designed and conducted a 10-week controlled clinical trial, in which children with NE received chiropractic or sham intervention. After the treatment, a significant reduction was observed in children's mean wet night frequency (from 9.1 to 6.7 nights/2 weeks) in chiropractic group. By contrast, the counterpart in sham intervention group did not change markedly (12.1 vs 12.2 nights/2 weeks) [60]. Van Poecke and his colleague found that the resolution rate within 1 year in children who received chiropractic was about 66.6% after analyzing the data of 33 patient records [61].

5. New about diagnostic and treatment

Enuretic bladder capacity is a big issue discussed in some recent research. Researchers are more likely to use the reduction in maximum voiding volume (MVV) on bladder diary to determine the decreased nocturnal bladder capacity (NBC). However, it might be unreasonable because a study found the enuretic bladder capacity of enuresis children was significantly less than their daytime functional bladder capacity (FBC), while healthy children's NBC was the same as FBC [62]. Kim et al.'s study also showed that the proportion of NE children with small NBC and small MVV was quite different. The accuracy using decreased MVV to identify small NBC is only medium to low [63]. Another study performed by Borg et al. measured the difference in diaper weight between the early part and the later part of the night, as the enuretic bladder capacity, in MNE children with normal MVV, and found that 82% of children had less bladder capacity than MVV during enuresis, even less than 65% of expected bladder capacity [64]. These studies indicate that although small MVV can be used to determine the reduction of FBC, it cannot assess accurately NBC or enuretic bladder capacity. If pediatricians manage MNE children with normal MVV with desmopressin following the ICCS guidelines, these children may still experience nocturnal enuresis due to a mismatch between bladder capacity and urine volume at night. Therefore, a new method for assessing NBC and enuretic bladder capacity needs to be explored.

Barroso et al. assessed the efficacy of a new device, which is the combination of alarm and electrical stimulation to the pelvic floor muscles, for NE. This device presented an advantage that helps children to achieve no wet beds during the period of treatment. On the one hand, pelvic floor muscle contraction induced by electrical stimulus may cause an increased urethral closure pressure, which allows children to keep dry during nighttime. On the other hand, alarm would also be triggered by the humidity sensor, and children would be waked to void [65]. This device needs more trials to determine its effectiveness and safety. Additionally, there was an intelligent autonomous alarm using ultrasound and smartphone ML techniques raised in 2019. It could monitor the bladder and trigger before the voiding desire. It also has the advantage to achieve totally dry bed during treatment [66].

6. Conclusions

Standard therapy should be applied to every child when he first visits the clinic. Then clinicians follow the diagnosis algorithm to distinguish MNE from NMNE and determine which subtype the child is. According to the ICCS's guideline [10], MNE children with normal nocturnal urine volume (normal or reduced MVV) should choose the alarm therapy. It is believed as the most effective single-therapy with the lower recurrence rate and has efficacy for most types of MNE, even NMNE. The addition of overlearning can reduce the relapse rate of alarm. Therefore, it is necessary to perform overlearning after the success of the alarm treatment. Complex behavioral therapies supplemented by alarm are more effective than alarm and can reduce the recurrence rate. It can be advised to families with better motivation and seeking for better efficacy. Desmopressin should be used for the treatment of MNE children with polyuria (normal or reduced MVV). To avoid relapse, the drug can be taken for a long time and then gradually reduced.

The guideline recommended small MVV and NP children to use combination therapy of alarm and desmopressin [10]. The addition of alarm can increase the long-term efficacy of desmopressin [37]. However, combination therapy seems not to reduce the number of children who do not achieve 14 consecutive dry nights compared with alarm alone [29], indicating that patients who do not have full response to these two therapies may be mostly overlapped.

For refractory NE, clinicians should reassess children's potential physiological malformations and neurogenic bladder diseases using MRI, urodynamics, cystoscopy, urography, etc. if necessary. After first-line treatment failure, children with detrusor overactivity or decreasing functional bladder capacity can choose anticholinergic drugs. Other children can choose tricyclic drugs, biofeedback therapy, electrical stimulation interventions, acupuncture, massage and so on, or a combination of first-line therapy and second-line therapy.

In summary, after meticulous diagnosis and assessment and appropriate treatment with sufficient evidence, most MNE children can get a great relief or even cure.

Author details

Bingying Zhou*, Jianxin Lu, Peiqi Shi and Yifang An
Guang'anmen Hospital, China Academy of Chinese Medical Sciences, Beijing, China

*Address all correspondence to: zhou1173538131@163.com

References

[1] Austin PF, Bauer SB, Bower W, et al. The standardization of terminology of lower urinary tract function in children and adolescents: Update report from the Standardization Committee of the International Children's Continence Society. Journal of Urology. 2014;**6**:1863-1865.e13. DOI: 10.1016/j.juro.2014.01.110

[2] Jain S, Bhatt GC. Advances in the management of primary monosymptomatic nocturnal enuresis in children. Paediatrics and International Child Health. 2016;**36**(1):7-14

[3] Bakhtiar K, Pournia Y, Ebrahimzadeh F, et al. Prevalence of nocturnal enuresis and its associated factors in primary school and preschool children of khorramabad in 2013. International Journal of Pediatrics. 2014:120686-120686

[4] Mejias SG, Ramphul K. Nocturnal enuresis in children from Santo Domingo, Dominican Republic: A questionnaire study of prevalence and risk factors. BMJ Paediatrics Open. 2018;**2**(1):e000311

[5] Hamed A, Yousf F, Hussein MM. Prevalence of nocturnal enuresis and related risk factors in school-age children in Egypt: An epidemiological study. World Journal of Urology. 2017;**35**(3):459-465

[6] Sarici H, Telli O, Ozgur BC, et al. Prevalence of nocturnal enuresis and its influence on quality of life in school-aged children. Journal of Pediatric Urology. 2016;**12**(3):159.e1-159.e6. DOI: 10.1016/j.jpurol.2015.11.011

[7] Gür E, Turhan P, Can G, et al. Enuresis: Prevalence, risk factors and urinary pathology among school children in Istanbul, Turkey. Pediatrics International: Official Journal of the Japan Pediatric Society. 2004;**46**(1):58-63

[8] Jarvelin M, Vikevainentervonen L, Moilanen I, et al. Enuresis in Seven-Year-Old Children. Acta Paediatrica. 1988;**77**(1):148-153

[9] Wen JG, Wang QW, Chen Y, et al. An epidemiological study of primary nocturnal enuresis in Chinese children and adolescents. European Urology. 2006;**49**(6):1107-1113

[10] Walle JV, Rittig S, Bauer S, et al. Practical consensus guidelines for the management of enuresis. European Journal of Pediatrics. 2012;**171**(6):971-983

[11] Dibianco JM, Morley C, Alomar O. Nocturnal enuresis: A topic review and institution experience. Avicenna Journal of Medicine. 2014;**4**:77

[12] Tekgul S, Nijman R, Hoebeke P, Canning D, Bower W, von Gontard A. Diagnosis and management of urinary incontinence in childhood.Report from the 4th International Consultation on Incontinence. Plymouth, UK: Health Publication Ltd; 2009. pp. 701-792

[13] Sorotzkin B. Nocturnal enuresis: Current perspectives. Clinical Psychology Review. 1984;**4**(3):293-315

[14] Neveus T, Eggert P, Evans J, et al. Evaluation of and treatment for monosymptomatic enuresis: A standardization document from the international children's continence society. The Journal of Urology. 2010;**183**(2):441-447

[15] Van Hoeck KJ, Bael A, Van Dessel E, et al. Do holding exercises or antimuscarinics increase maximum voided volume in monosymptomatic nocturnal enuresis? A randomized controlled trial in children. The Journal of Urology. 2007;**178**(5):2132-2136. DOI: 10.1016/j.juro.2007.07.051

[16] Caldwell PHY, Nankivell G, Sureshkumar P. Simple behavioural interventions for nocturnal enuresis in children. Cochrane Database of Systematic Reviews. 2013;(7):CD003637. DOI: 10.1002/14651858.CD003637.pub3

[17] Tkaczyk M, Maternik M, Krakowska A, et al. Evaluation of the effect of 3-month bladder basic advice in children with monosymptomatic nocturnal enuresis. Journal of Pediatric Urology. 2017;**13**(6):615.e1-615.e6. DOI: 10.1016/j.jpurol.2017.03.039

[18] Kroll P, Zachwieja J. The system of management nocturnal enuresis based on functional classification. Przegląd Lekarski. 2006;**63**:229-232

[19] Butler RJ, Redfern EJ, Holland P. Children's notions about enuresis and the implications for treatment. Scandinavian Journal of Urology and Nephrology. Supplementum. 1994;**163**:39-47

[20] van Dommelen P, Kamphuis M, van Leerdam FJ, et al. The short- and long-term effects of simple behavioral interventions for nocturnal enuresis in young children: A randomized controlled trial. The Journal of Pediatrics. 2009;**154**(5):662-666. DOI: 10.1016/j.jpeds.2008.12.001

[21] Hofmeester I, Kollen BJ, Steffens MG, et al. Predictors for a positive outcome of adapted clinical dry bed training in adolescents and adults with enuresis. Neurourology and Urodynamics. 2016;**35**(8):1006-1010. DOI: 10.1002/nau.22869

[22] Brown ML, Pope AW, Brown EJ. Treatment of primary nocturnal enuresis in children: A review. Child: Care, Health and Development. 2011;**37**(2):153-160. DOI: 10.1111/j.1365-2214.2010.01146.x

[23] Glazener CMA, Evans JHC, Peto RE. Complex behavioural and educational interventions for nocturnal enuresis in children. Cochrane Database of Systematic Reviews. 2004;(1):CD004668. DOI: 10.1002/14651858.CD004668

[24] van Londen A, van Londen-Barentsen MW, van Son MJ, et al. Arousal training for children suffering from nocturnal enuresis: A 2 1/2 year follow-up. Behaviour Research and Therapy. 1993;**31**(6):613-615

[25] Van Kampen M, Bogaert G, Feys H, et al. High initial efficacy of full-spectrum therapy for nocturnal enuresis in children and adolescents. BJU International. 2002;**90**(1):84-87

[26] Hoekx L, Vermandel A, Wyndaele JJ. Functional bladder capacity after bladder biofeedback predicts long-term outcome in children with nocturnal enuresis. Scandinavian Journal of Urology and Nephrology. 2003;**37**(2):120-123. DOI: 10.1080/00365590310008848

[27] Kajbafzadeh AM, Sharifi-Rad L, Mozafarpour S, et al. Efficacy of transcutaneous interferential electrical stimulation in treatment of children with primary nocturnal enuresis: A randomized clinical trial. Pediatric Nephrology. 2015;**30**(7):1139-1145. DOI: 10.1007/s00467-014-3039-5

[28] Abd El-Moghny SM, El-Din MS, El Shemy SA. Effectiveness of intra-anal biofeedback and electrical stimulation in the treatment of children with refractory monosymptomatic nocturnal enuresis: A comparative randomized controlled trial. International Neurourology Journal. 2018;**22**(4):295-304. DOI: 10.5213/inj.1836142.071

[29] Glazener CMA, Evans JHC, Peto RE. Alarm interventions for nocturnal enuresis in children. Cochrane Database of Systematic Reviews. 2005;(2):CD002911. DOI: 10.1002/14651858.CD002911.pub2

[30] Tsuji S, Suruda C, Kimata T, et al. The effect of family assistance to wake children with monosymptomatic enuresis in alarm therapy: A pilot study. The Journal of Urology. 2018;**199**(4):1056-1060. DOI: 10.1016/j.juro.2017.11.072

[31] Apos E, Schuster S, Reece J, et al. Enuresis management in children: Retrospective clinical audit of 2861 cases treated with practitioner-assisted bell-and-pad alarm. Journal of Pediatrics. 2018;**193**:211-216. DOI: 10.1016/j.jpeds.2017.09.086

[32] Kosilov KV, Geltser BI, Loparev SA, et al. The optimal duration of alarm therapy use in children with primary monosymptomatic nocturnal enuresis. Journal of Pediatric Urology. 2018;**14**(5):447.e1-447.e6. DOI: 10.1016/j.jpurol.2018.03.021

[33] Hyuga T, Nakamura S, Kawai S, et al. Evaluation of the effectiveness of a short-term treatment and repeat treatment of nocturnal enuresis using an enuresis alarm. Urology. 2017;**105**:153-156. DOI: 10.1016/j.urology.2017.01.005

[34] Schulz-Juergensen S, Langguth A, Eggert P. Effect of alarm therapy on conditioning of central reflex control in nocturnal enuresis: Pilot study on changes in prepulse inhibition (PPI). Pediatric Nephrology. 2014;**29**(7):1209-1213. DOI: 10.1007/s00467-014-2756-0

[35] Hvistendahl GM, Kamperis K, Rawashdeh YF, et al. The effect of alarm treatment on the functional bladder capacity in children with monosymptomatic nocturnal enuresis. Journal of Urology. 2004;**6**(Pt 2):2611-2614

[36] Schulz-Juergensen S, Rieger M, Schaefer J, et al. Effect of 1-desamino-8-D-arginine vasopressin on prepulse inhibition of startle supports a central etiology of primary monosymptomatic enuresis. The Journal of Pediatrics. 2007;**151**(6):571-574. DOI: 10.1016/j.jpeds.2007.05.024

[37] Glazener CMA, Evans JHC. Desmopressin for nocturnal enuresis in children. Cochrane Database of Systematic Reviews. 2002;(3):CD002112. DOI: 10.1002/14651858.CD002112

[38] Rittig S, Schaumburg H, Schmidt F, et al. Long-term home studies of water balance in patients with nocturnal enuresis. Scandinavian Journal of Urology and Nephrology. 1997;**183**:25-26; discussion 26-7

[39] Hamano S, Yamanishi T, Igarashi T, et al. Functional bladder capacity as predictor of response to desmopressin and retention control training in monosymptomatic nocturnal enuresis. European Urology. 2000;**37**(6):718-722. DOI: 10.1159/000020224

[40] Yeung CK, Sreedhar B, Leung VT, et al. Ultrasound bladder measurements in patients with primary nocturnal enuresis: A urodynamic and treatment outcome correlation. Journal of Urology. 2004;**6**(Pt 2):2589-2594

[41] Wolfish NM, Barkin J, Gorodzinsky F, et al. The Canadian enuresis study and evaluation—Short- and long-term safety and efficacy of an oral desmopressin preparation. Scandinavian Journal of Urology and Nephrology. 2003;**37**(1):22-27. DOI: 10.1080/00365590310008631

[42] Caldwell PHY, Sureshkumar P, Wong WCF. Tricyclic and related drugs for nocturnal enuresis in children. Cochrane Database of Systematic Reviews. 2016;(1):CD002117. DOI: 10.1002/14651858.CD002117.pub2

[43] Neveus T. Reboxetine in therapy-resistant enuresis: Results

and pathogenetic implications. Scandinavian Journal of Urology and Nephrology. 2006;**40**(1):31-34. DOI: 10.1080/00365590500407803

[44] Lundmark E, Stenberg A, Hagglof B, et al. Reboxetine in therapy-resistant enuresis: A randomized placebo-controlled study. Journal of Pediatric Urology. 2016;**12**(6):397.e1-397.e5. DOI: 10.1016/j.jpurol.2016.04.048

[45] Kwak KW, Lee YS, Park KH, et al. Efficacy of desmopressin and enuresis alarm as first and second line treatment for primary monosymptomatic nocturnal enuresis: Prospective randomized crossover study. Journal of Urology. 2010;**184**(6):2521-2526. DOI: 10.1016/j.juro.2010.08.041

[46] Butler RJ, Holland P, Gasson S, et al. Exploring potential mechanisms in alarm treatment for primary nocturnal enuresis. Scandinavian Journal of Urology and Nephrology. 2007;**41**(5):407-413. DOI: 10.1080/00365590701571506

[47] Tempest H, Reynard J, Bryant RJ, et al. Acupuncture in urological practice—A survey of urologists in England. Complementary Therapies in Medicine. 2011;**19**(1):27-31. DOI: 10.1016/j.ctim.2010.10.001

[48] Bjorkstrom G, Hellstrom AL, Andersson S. Electro-acupuncture in the treatment of children with monosymptomatic nocturnal enuresis. Scandinavian Journal of Urology and Nephrology. 2000;**34**(1):21-26

[49] Honjo H, Kawauchi A, Ukimura O, et al. Treatment of monosymptomatic nocturnal enuresis by acupuncture: A preliminary study. International Journal of Urology. 2002;**9**(12):672-676

[50] Huang T, Shu X, Huang YS, et al. Complementary and miscellaneous interventions for nocturnal enuresis in children. Cochrane Database of Systematic Reviews. 2011;(12):CD005230. DOI: 10.1002/14651858.CD005230.pub2

[51] Bower WF, Diao M, Tang JL, et al. Acupuncture for nocturnal enuresis in children: A systematic review and exploration of rationale. Neurourology and Urodynamics. 2005;**24**(3):267-272. DOI: 10.1002/nau.20108

[52] Lv ZT, Song W, Wu J, et al. Efficacy of acupuncture in children with nocturnal enuresis: A systematic review and meta-analysis of randomized controlled trials. Evidence-based Complementary and Alternative Medicine. 2015;**2015**:320701. DOI: 10.1155/2015/320701

[53] Minni B, Capozza N, Creti G, et al. Bladder instability and enuresis treated by acupuncture and electro-therapeutics: Early urodynamic observations. Acupuncture & Electro-Therapeutics Research. 1990;**151**(1):19-25

[54] Yang J, Yang Y, Wang CH, et al. Effect of arginine vasopressin on acupuncture analgesia in the rat. Peptides. 2009;**302**(2):241-247. DOI: 10.1016/j.peptides.2008.10.013

[55] Culbert TP, Banez GA. Wetting the bed: Integrative approaches to nocturnal enuresis. Explore (New York, N.Y.). 2008;**4**(3):215-220. DOI: 10.1016/j.explore.2008.02.014

[56] Sharifi H, Minaie MB, Qasemzadeh MJ, et al. Topical use of *Matricaria recutita* L (chamomile) oil in the treatment of monosymptomatic enuresis in children: A double-blind randomized controlled trial. Journal Evidence-Based Complementary and Alternative Medicine. 2017;**22**(1):12-17. DOI: 10.1177/2156587215608989

[57] Bartocci C, Lucentini M. Acupuncture and micro-massage in the treatment of idiopathic nocturnal

enuresis. Minerva Medica. 1981;**72**(33):2237

[58] Yuksek MS, Erdem AF, Atalay C, et al. Acupressure versus oxybutinin in the treatment of enuresis. Journal of International Medical Research. 2003;**31**(6):552-556. DOI: 10.1177/147323000303100611

[59] Leboeuf C, Brown P, Herman A, et al. Chiropractic care of children with nocturnal enuresis: A prospective outcome study. Journal of Manipulative and Physiological Therapeutics. 1991;**14**(2):110-115

[60] Reed WR, Beavers S, Reddy SK, et al. Chiropractic management of primary nocturnal enuresis. Journal of Manipulative and Physiological Therapeutics. 1994;**17**(9):596-600

[61] van Poecke AJ, Cunliffe C. Chiropractic treatment for primary nocturnal enuresis: A case series of 33 consecutive patients. Journal of Manipulative and Physiological Therapeutics. 2009;**32**(8):675-681. DOI: 10.1016/j.jmpt.2009.08.019

[62] Kawauchi A, Tanaka Y, Naito Y, et al. Bladder capacity at the time of enuresis. Urology. 2003;**61**(5):1016-1018

[63] Kim JM, Park JW, Lee CS. Evaluation of nocturnal bladder capacity and nocturnal urine volume in nocturnal enuresis. Journal of Pediatric Urology. 2014;**10**(3):559-563. DOI: 10.1016/j.jpurol.2013.11.020

[64] Borg B, Kamperis K, Olsen LH, et al. Evidence of reduced bladder capacity during nighttime in children with monosymptomatic nocturnal enuresis. Journal of Pediatric Urology. 2018;**14**(2):160.e1-160.e6. DOI: 10.1016/j.jpurol.2017.09.021

[65] Barroso U Jr, Lordelo P, Teles A, et al. New device and new concept for treating nocturnal enuresis: Preliminary results of a phase one study. Journal of Pediatric Urology. 2014;**10**(6):1273-1276. DOI: 10.1016/j.jpurol.2014.06.023

[66] Kuru K, Ansell D, Jones M, et al. Feasibility study of intelligent autonomous determination of the bladder voiding need to treat bedwetting using ultrasound and smartphone ML techniques: Intelligent autonomous treatment of bedwetting. Medical & Biological Engineering & Computing. 2019;**57**(5):1079-1097. DOI: 10.1007/s11517-018-1942-9

Chapter 6

Historical Perspective and Innovations in Penile Urethroplasty

Francisco E. Martins, Pedro Simoes de Oliveira and Natalia M. Martins

Abstract

Penile urethral strictures are common and impact on quality of life and healthcare costs. Management of penile urethral strictures is complex and depends on the physical characteristics of the stricture. Contemporary studies show no difference between urethral dilation and internal urethrotomy in terms of long-term outcomes. Overall, long-term success rates range from 20 to 30%. However, their recurrence rate is greater for men with longer strictures, penile urethral strictures, multiple strictures, presence of infection, or history of prior procedures, which make them less cost-effective. Surgical urethroplasty is associated with higher long-term success rates, averaging from 85 to 90%, mostly in virgin or noncomplex cases. Historically, modern urethral reconstruction has evolved from 1950s with the revolutionary introduction of Johanson's technique for staged urethral reconstruction. Since then, many techniques have been developed and employed for urethroplasty, depending on the location, length, and character of the stricture. Successful management of urethral strictures requires detailed knowledge of anatomy, pathophysiology, proper patient selection, and reconstructive techniques.

Keywords: anterior urethra, urethral stricture, urethroplasty, penile

1. Introduction

Urethral strictures have been common since ancient times. Knowledge was gathered about the treatment of urethral stricture disease by ancient Egyptians and other civilizations more than two millennia ago. Nonetheless, little has changed until about 60 years ago. Since then, the management of urethral strictures, including the penile urethral segment, has been in continuous and rapid evolution. Although various reconstructive techniques are available for the treatment of penile urethral stricture, no single technique has been identified as the method of choice. An understanding of the penile urethral anatomy is important for the diagnosis and treatment of penile urethral stricture disease.

Urethral strictures, in general, are associated with significant impact on patients' quality of life. Penile urethral strictures, in particular, due to their exposed anatomic location and their surgical treatment, may cause significant impact on patients' sexual function and perception of (un)satisfactory penile cosmesis.

The anatomical and physical characteristics of the penile urethra are associated with additional challenges when compared to other urethral locations, especially due to its unsuitability for anastomotic repair and its relatively thinner corpus spongiosum. The choice of penile urethroplasty technique is largely influenced by etiology, location, length of the stricture, as well as prior surgical treatments. There are a number of challenges and controversies in the surgical reconstruction of penile urethral strictures, such as the use of grafts vs. flaps, use of skin vs. oral mucosa graft (OMG) tissue for augmentation or substitution techniques, the most appropriate indications for a single or a staged (at times, multiple) reconstruction, and, lastly, the management of particularly complex cases such as panurethral stricture disease and hypospadias "cripples" to achieve the best possible outcome.

Although penile urethral strictures can be managed by any of the above-mentioned procedures individually, they can also be more adequately treated by a combined approach. Among the various procedures available for treating urethral stricture, one-stage buccal mucosal graft urethroplasty is the current standard practice. The selection of technique for penile urethroplasty for an individual patient largely depends not only on the expertise of the surgeon but also upon the stricture's etiology, pathological characteristics, and location. Therefore, contemporary reconstructive urologists working in this field should be aware of, and permanently keep themselves updated on, the numerous surgical techniques required to deal with any condition of the urethra that might surface at the time of surgery.

This review provides a brief update of the options for the surgical reconstruction of different types and sites of penile urethral stricture as well as discussing current controversies, innovations, and possible future research in urethral reconstruction of the penile urethra.

2. Anatomical considerations

Classically, the anterior urethra is divided, at the level of the penoscrotal junction inferiorly and the suspensory ligament superiorly, into bulbar and penile segments, the penile part consisting of the external meatus, fossa navicularis, and the penile shaft urethra. The penile urethra extends from the distal margin of the bulbospongiosus (or penoscrotal junction) to the external meatus. The bulbar (proximal) segment is the shorter of the two and is located in the midline between both the penile crural and the cavernosal bodies. The penile urethra (distal segment of the anterior urethra), also called pendulous, lies in a dorsal groove between the two corpora cavernosa and extends from the penoscrotal junction to the tip of the glans penis. It is surrounded in its full length by the corpus spongiosum; it is mobile and stretches during penile erection; and its length varies according to the penile length. The caliber of the anterior urethral lumen is relatively uniform, widening distally to form the fossa navicularis, and narrowing again to end at the external meatus (**Figure 1**).

Histologically, the penile (distal anterior) urethra is surrounded by five tissue layers: urethral epithelium and lamina propria (urethral mucosa), corpus spongiosum, tunica albuginea, and Buck's fascia [1]. Most of the penile shaft urethra is lined by a stratified and pseudostratified columnar epithelium, except for the distal penile urethra, including the fossa navicularis, which is lined by ciliated stratified columnar epithelium or stratified nonkeratinizing squamous epithelium. The lamina propria of the penile urethra is a fibroconnective tissue with elastic fibers and scattered, longitudinally oriented smooth muscle fibers. Multiple mucus-secreting glands drain into the anterior urethral lumen, known as Cowper's glands in the bulbar urethra and Littre's glands in the penile urethra.

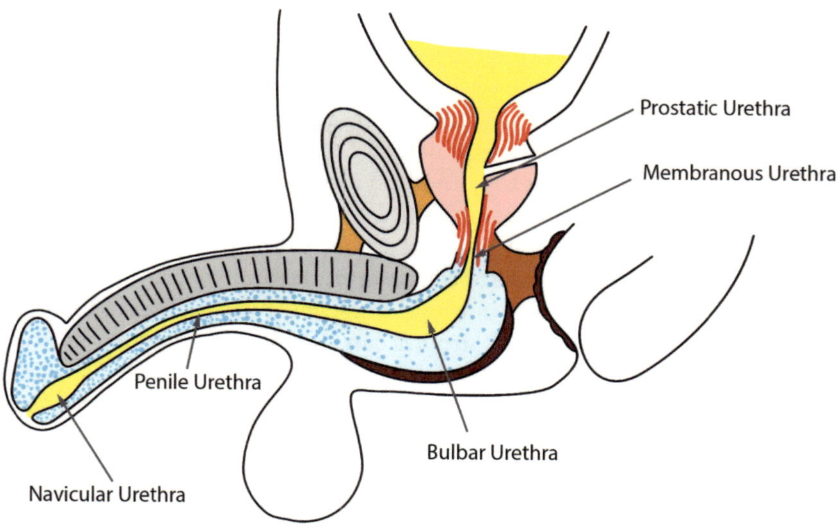

Figure 1.
Sagittal sectional view of the male urethra. The areas in blue and yellow represent the corpus spongiosum and lumen of the anterior urethra, respectively. The penile urethra extends distally from the penoscrotal junction or pubourethral ligaments (reproduced with permission from Dr. Enzo Palminteri).

The anterior urethra obtains its blood supply from the first of three penile branches of the internal pudendal artery, which in turn is a branch of the internal iliac artery. The internal pudendal artery travels through the Alcock canal and gives the inferior rectal artery, posterior scrotal artery and perineal artery, and then terminates as the common penile artery. Three branches arise from the common penile artery: the paired urethral or, most commonly, bulbourethral arteries that pierce the perineal body at a posterolateral location and supply the urethra, spongiosum, and the glans. The other branches are the paired cavernosal arteries that pierce the penile hilum to travel in the center of the erectile tissue, and the deep dorsal penile artery that travel between the crura and beneath the pubic bone to run under the Buck's fascia sending multiple circumflex branches to the corpus spongiosum and terminal branches to the glans penis, thus providing in a retrograde fashion a dual blood supply to the corpus spongiosum and urethra. It also sends cavernosal branches to contribute to the hemodynamics of the erection (**Figure 2A** and **B**). The venous

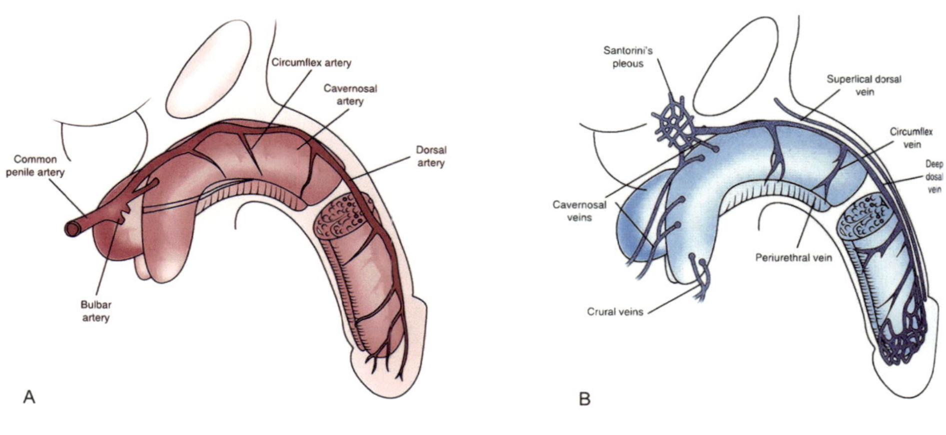

Figure 2.
Schematic illustration of vascularization of the penis and urethra: (A) arterial blood supply and (B) venous blood drainage.

drainage is through the emissary veins into the circumflex branches of the deep dorsal penile vein as well as through the urethral and bulbar veins into the internal pudendal vein. The anterior urethra is innervated by the urethrobulbar nerve, a branch of the perineal nerve derived from the pudendal nerve. The bulbocavernosus nerve, which is a branch of the pudendal nerve, gives off two branches that penetrate the rhabdosphincter at the three and nine o'clock positions. The pudendal nerve, gathering fibers from the second, third and fourth sacral spinal nerve, is both motor to the urethral rhabdosphincter and sensory to the urethra and glans penis (**Figure 3**). The lymphatic drainage of the anterior urethra is via the superficial and deep inguinal nodes, whereas the lymphatic drainage of the more proximal (the bulbar, membranous, and prostatic) urethra can take three routes: to the external iliac nodes, to the obturator and internal iliac nodes, or to the presacral nodes [2].

Understanding the penile anatomy and, in particular, the penile skin arterial blood supply is an important resource for penile urethral surgical reconstruction. The penis is covered with an elastic layer of skin that has no subcuticular adipose tissue: the dartos fascia, a layer of loose areolar subcutaneous connective tissue in the penis and scrotum. It lies immediately beneath the penile skin, allowing the skin to move freely over the shaft of the penis and is contiguous with Colles fascia in the perineum. The dartos, also with no adipose tissue, slides freely over the underlying Buck's fascia and is an extension of Scarpa's fascia of the abdominal wall, carrying superficial nerves, lymphatics, and blood vessels, which make this fascia extremely useful in bringing blood supply and preventing fistulation in urethral reconstruction. Beneath the dartos fascia lies the Buck's fascia, which surrounds the tunica albuginea of the two corpora cavernosa and the corpus spongiosum.

The development of fasciocutaneous penile skin island flaps, either as a vertical flap (as in Orandi flap) or as a circular transverse flap (as in McAninch/Quartey flap), takes advantage of the natural anatomical, relatively avascular cleavage planes between the skin and the dartos fascia and another between the dartos fascia and Buck's fascia.

The blood supply to the penile skin and anterior scrotal wall comes from the external pudendal arteries, whereas the inferior and posterior aspect of the scrotum

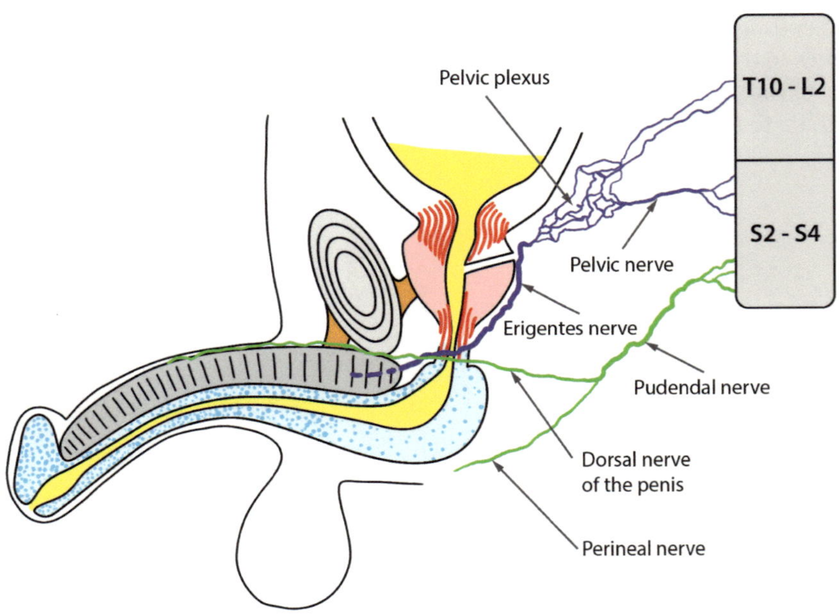

Figure 3.
Schematic illustration of autonomic and somatic innervation of the penis and urethra (reproduced with permission from Dr. Enzo Palminteri).

derives its blood supply from the posterior scrotal arteries, which are branches of the perineal artery, which in turn is a further branch of the internal pudendal artery (**Figure 4**). The superficial/superior branches of the external pudendal artery travel from medially and across the femoral triangle and within Scarpa's fascia to enter the base of the penis. After giving off anterior scrotal branches, they arborize to form an arterial network within the dartos fascia. Also, at the base of the penis, branches from the axial penile artery form a subdermal plexus to supply the distal penile skin and prepuce. Because the communicating vessels between the subcutaneous and subdermal arterial plexuses are minimal, a relatively avascular plane can be developed between the dartos and Buck's fascia. This fascial plexus, that is considered axial, is the true blood supply to the penile island skin flaps used in urethroplasty and, therefore, they can be mobilized widely and transposed aggressively and reliably.

The venous drainage of the penis includes the superficial dorsal vein, the deep dorsal vein, and the crural veins. The superficial dorsal vein drains the skin of the penis and empties into the superficial external pudendal vein and then into the saphenous vein. The deep dorsal vein begins at the base of the glans and retro coronal area and then travels deep to the Buck's fascia between the paired deep dorsal arteries. Along its course, it receives circumflex veins from the spongiosum until it passes under the pubic bone to join the periprostatic venous complex. The cavernosal veins drain into a subtunical venous plexus; then through emissary veins, they join the circumflex veins, which in turn empty into the crural vein and the periprostatic plexus or the internal pudendal veins. The lymphatic drainage of the penis is primarily to the superficial inguinal nodes.

A detailed understanding of the anatomy of the anterior urethra is a critical prerequisite for the accurate diagnosis and successful management of urethral strictures.

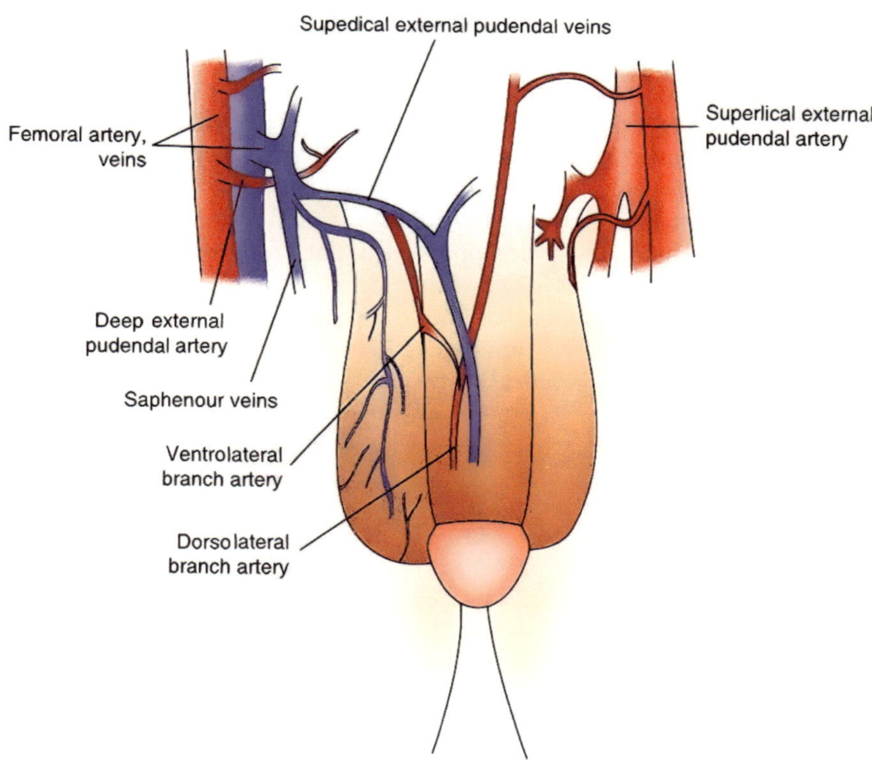

Figure 4.
Schematic illustration of the superficial arterial supply and venous drainage of the penis and scrotum.

3. Etiology

The etiology of contemporary urethral stricture disease involves a traumatic, iatrogenic, inflammatory, and idiopathic origin [3, 4]. Pathophysiology differs with age. The major causes of anterior urethral stricture in children are more likely to be trauma, mainly straddle injury, and complications from hypospadias surgery. Congenital and idiopathic strictures may also occur in children. In adult patients, most urethral strictures have an iatrogenic origin, mainly traumatic catheterization or transurethral manipulation or instrumentation. In the <10-year-old age group, strictures are mainly localized in the penile urethra, whereas in the >10-year-old age group, the bulbar urethra is the most common location [5].

In the past, inflammatory urethral strictures were predominantly associated with gonococcal urethritis, which has been effectively eradicated with penicillin-based antimicrobial agents. However, the emergence of resistant strains of *Neisseria gonorrhoeae* may be responsible for resurgence in these cases. Lichen sclerosus (LS, also and erroneously known as balanitis xerotica obliterans) is another inflammatory and challenging cause of urethral stricture disease, which usually involves genital skin, often progressing to panurethral stricture disease, and is associated with comorbidities, such as diabetes and obesity, which may aggravate surgical treatment [6, 7].

Stricture etiology is of particular significance in the penile urethra, as they tend to be more diffuse in nature (averaging 6.1 cm), especially if associated with LS, and shorter in the bulbar urethra (averaging 3.1 cm). Urethral strictures can be classified by their most common urethral location. Strictures involving the external meatus and fossa navicularis are predominantly inflammatory and iatrogenic in origin in 33–47% [3]. In the series reported by Fenton et al., globally, the etiology of anterior urethral strictures was idiopathic in 34%, iatrogenic in 32%, inflammatory in 20%, and traumatic in 14% [3].

Iatrogenic strictures are typically associated with instrumentation, such as transurethral resection, prolonged catheterization, and cystoscopy, totaling 90% of all penile strictures. Prior hypospadias repair and radical prostatectomy contributed to 6.3 and 3.2%, respectively [3, 8]. Such strictures are mainly the result of an ischemic injury secondary to traumatic urethral manipulation or instrumentation, particularly when a large bore catheter or resectoscope is used. Therefore, whenever relatively prolonged catheterization is necessary, smaller caliber/Fr catheters are recommended. For more extended periods of time, a suprapubic catheter is a better option.

Malignant strictures should be approached in a different clinical context and most likely require mutilating radical surgery.

Urethral dilatation
Internal urethrotomy
Laser urethrotomy
Grafts
Flaps
Combination of grafts and flaps
One-stage urethroplasty
Staged urethroplasty

Table 1.
Management options for penile urethral strictures.

4. Diagnostic evaluation

Clinical evaluation: the diagnosis of penile urethral strictures, like any other type of stricture, regardless of location, is based on a suggestive clinical history and physical examination. The main symptoms are related to obstructive voiding or urinary tract infection, or both. Some patients may less often present with urinary retention. Weak stream, incomplete bladder emptying, and a hyperactive bladder are usually the most prevalent complaints of patients with anterior urethral stricture [9]. If questioned carefully, most patients who present in chronic retention may state that their symptoms have been present for a long time, which they have tolerated fairly well and, therefore, have been neglected. In some occasions, the diagnosis is brought up to the urologist's attention because of difficult urethral catheterization for any reason, often in the operating theater before an operation that requires routine urethral catheterization. In about 1.3%, renal failure is the initial presentation of a urethral stricture [9].

Any relevant past history of urethral instrumentation, hypospadias surgery, and genital trauma should be obtained. Obstructive voiding symptoms should be assessed with a validated questionnaire. Presence of risk factors and comorbidities that may provoke ischemia or impair wound healing should be probed for. These include obesity, diabetes mellitus, severe peripheral vascular disease, cigarette smoking, long-distance bicycle riding, horseback riding, and sexually transmitted infections.

Physical examination should include palpation of the penile shaft for nodules or dense urethral scarring or constriction. The urethral meatus should be examined for narrowing and the surrounding glans for signs of LS. The penis should be examined to assess whether the patient has been circumcised, or there is sufficient shaft skin to allow development of a penile skin flap. The bladder should be assessed for potential detrusor hypocontractility, distention, and presence of an abdominal scar from a previous suprapubic cystostomy.

Uroflowmetry: this test provides a quantitative estimate of the severity of obstruction. A flattened, "en plateau" voiding pattern along with elevated postvoid residual urine volume signals the degree of urethral narrowing and efficiency of voiding and bladder emptying (**Figure 5**). More formal urodynamic studies (pressure-flow studies) are rarely indicated or necessary, except for complex cases or when the anatomic location of obstruction is needed in presence of concomitant prostatic obstruction.

Radiographic contrast studies: contrast studies of the urethra are the cornerstone of the imaging diagnosis. The combination of dynamic retrograde urethrogram and voiding cystourethrogram allows accurate assessment of stricture length and location (**Figure 6**). Dynamic retrograde urethrogram has been rated the gold standard of urethral stricture evaluation with a specificity and sensitivity of 90% [10].

Ultrasonography/sonourethrography: ultrasonography has a limited role in the evaluation of the male urethra. It may be useful to detect concomitant lesions such as calculus, trauma-induced soft tissue injury, or Peyronie's plaques that may coexist with urethral stricture disease. Sonourethrography, introduced in the mid-1980s, was reported to be a more accurate tool for the diagnosis and characterization of strictures, particularly in the bulbar urethra [11]. In addition to providing accurate information of the urethral stricture characteristics, sonourethrography allows assessment of the health and integrity of the soft tissues surrounding the strictured urethra. This modality represents an adjunct to contrast-enhanced studies and can increase the accuracy of anterior stricture length and spongiofibrosis as well as the inner diameter of the urethral lumen and, thus, improve surgical planning [12].

Endoscopy: endoscopic evaluation of a urethral stricture has a limited role as it allows only the identification of the most distal portion of the urethra. It does not determine

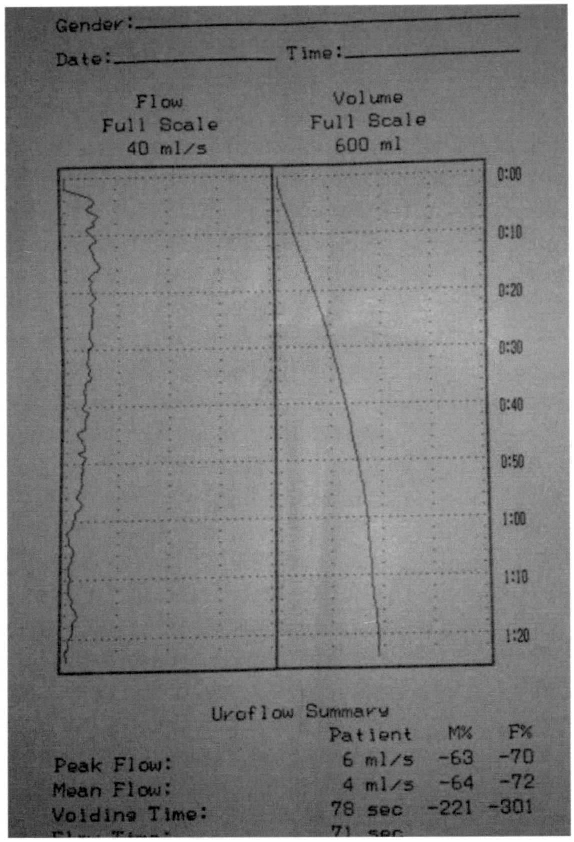

Figure 5.
"En plateau" obstructive uroflow in a patient with anterior urethral stricture.

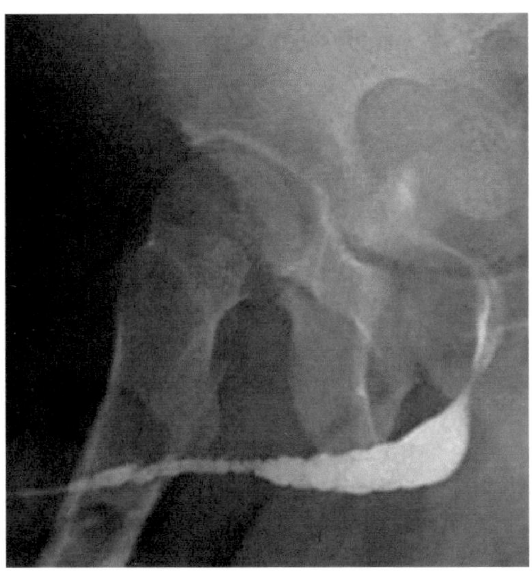

Figure 6.
Retrograde urethrogram of long, irregular, "saw-toothed" penile urethral stricture typical of lichen sclerosus.

the length of the stricture nor can it assess the proximal stricture extremity and the corresponding proximal urethra. However, it may help to determine the amount of distal urethral elasticity, or when the insertion of a guide-wire through the stricture is necessary or deemed safe, or in a rare case of suspicion of urethral carcinoma.

5. Preoperative planning and intraoperative decision-making

Any appropriate treatment plan needs accurate identification of the stricture characteristics: location, length, depth, and thickness of fibrotic tissue (spongiofibrosis). It is critical that both the proximal and distal ends of a urethral stricture are completely and accurately assessed with endoscopy and bougienage during reconstruction as to not miss any diseased segment of the urethra. Both patient and urethral reconstructive surgeons must understand completely the goal(s) of treatment before a decision is made. The decision to choose urethroplasty over another approach to a specific urethral stricture depends on patient expectations, goals, and comorbidities. In elderly or frail patients, an expectant or conservative management is more likely to be offered. Therefore, treatment options and their individual potential outcomes in terms of cure, or simply palliation, and complications should be carefully discussed with the patients and their family. On the other hand, urethral reconstructive surgeons need to keep themselves updated and abreast regarding the vast array of treatment options and their precise and specific indications and, therefore, should be flexible enough to intraoperatively adapt and/or adopt a different strategy for a specific scenario, which was not anticipated preoperatively. Thus, it is only legitimate and ethical to embark on urethral reconstruction if one can master and offer the patient all necessary surgical options to treat his specific urethral problem. It is very important to bear in mind that the penile urethra is the most exposed segment of the male urethra, and any surgical procedure or technique should achieve not only a satisfactory functional outcome but also a cosmetic one.

6. Management options

The key techniques include mainly urethral dilatation, endoscopic urethrotomy, anastomotic repairs (rarely in the penile urethra), substitution repairs (ventral, dorsal, double-faced), free grafts of skin (full thickness and split thickness skin), oral mucosa, lingual mucosa, bladder mucosa, retroauricular skin (Wolf's graft), and skin flap repairs (circumferential, longitudinal and variants) from penile and (less commonly) scrotal skin, as well as the use of adjunctive maneuvers such as the use of advancement flaps for additional blood supply or defect coverage (**Table 1**).

Urethral dilatation: several methods for urethral dilatation exist: dilatation with a balloon, filiform and followers, urethral sounds (metallic or nonmetallic), or self-catheter dilatation. Urethral dilatation is carried out by gradual progressive stretching of the urethral lumen to a maximal diameter of 24 Fr. However, if performed aggressively, it will lead to further urethral trauma and scarring. It should be regarded as a palliative procedure and rarely as a curative one. It is mainly indicated in very select cases of strictures of the external meatus and fossa navicularis. It should be avoided in patients with LS as it often worsens the inflammatory process. Repeat dilatation should be avoided as it does not treat the underlying dense spongiofibrosis associated with more complex strictures.

Internal urethrotomy: also called direct vision internal urethrotomy (DVIU), it was first described by Sachse [13]. It consists of a cold-knife incision of the scar tissue allowing its release and healing of the underlying tissue by secondary epithelialization around a urethral catheter and thereby increasing the diameter of the urethral lumen. Apparently, only superficial strictures benefit from this treatment option when the incision is carried out through all thickness of the scar. Its success depends mostly on stricture length and degree of spongiofibrosis [14, 15]. It is best indicated for short strictures (<1.5 cm in length). Heyns et al. have suggested that if the stricture has not recurred within the first 3 months after a single DVIU (or dilatation), the stricture-free rate is 50–60% for up to 4 years of follow-up evaluation [16]. Recurrence rates vary in the penile and bulbar urethra: 84 and 58%, respectively [17]. Like dilatation, repeat urethrotomy is known to be associated with worse outcomes [15–18]. The failure rates of these minimally invasive strategies are poor and well documented, ranging from 9% after 1–3 years of follow-up [18]. At ≥4 years, the chance of stricture-free status is nearly 0% [19]. Open urethral reconstruction should be considered in case of recurrence after these minimally invasive attempts, unless the patient prefers intermittent self-catheterization as a chronic treatment plan. Nonetheless, despite the limitation of these minimally invasive procedures, they may become more useful if new generations of currently experimental modalities for scar modulation prove successful [20].

Laser urethrotomy: it utilizes several types of lasers, including CO_2, argon, potassium titanyl phosphate (KTP), neodymium-doped yttrium aluminum garnet (Nd:YAG), holmium, and excimer lasers. They use different technologies and different depths of tissue penetration.

A meta-analysis of outcomes and complications of laser versus cold-knife urethrotomy compared unfavorably regarding laser: 12 versus 6.5%, respectively [21]. Laser urethrotomy may look appealing for the anterior urethra but with no definitive benefit over cold-knife urethrotomy.

Grafts: excision and primary reanastomosis, onlay grafting, and the use of flaps have been used for anterior urethral reconstruction. However, anastomotic urethroplasty rarely has a place in the penile shaft urethra due to the high risk of penile chordee or curvature, which impacts on erectile function and cosmesis. In the penile urethra, graft urethroplasty is traditionally used as it does not cause urethral tension. Several types of tissue can be used as onlay/inlay grafts: skin (full-thickness or split-thickness grafts), bladder mucosa, oral mucosa (buccal, labial, or lingual), and rectal mucosa. Historically, preputial skin grafts were the mainstay of grafting material until oral mucosa became popularized in the early 1990s [22, 23]. The crucial factor for grafting success is that the local tissue must have a healthy blood supply for normal graft taking. Single-stage graft urethroplasty uses the rich blood supply of spongiosal tissue ventrally or dorsally to support the graft, with overall success rates approaching 75–90% in the penile urethra, depending on stricture length [24, 25]. Little is found in the literature regarding both bladder epithelial grafts and rectal mucosal grafts, mainly due to lack of data about the process of take of these grafts.

Oral mucosal graft is currently the graft of choice, owing to their short harvest time, easy harvest technique, and the physical characteristics including resistance, durability, immunogenic properties, excellent vascularity, hairlessness, low oral morbidity, concealed donor site and high success rates [24, 25]. For these reasons, over the past 20 years, oral mucosal grafts have shown better handling characteristics and long-term stricture-free outcomes, and have replaced both penile skin grafts and flaps. However, patients with long and complex urethral abnormalities or with contraindications to oral mucosal graft use, such as those with leukoplakia, systemic skin disease of the oral cavity or history of chronic tobacco chewing may still necessitate split or full thickness skin grafts.

One controversy in anterior urethral grafting is related to dorsal or ventral placement of the graft on the urethra. Some urethral surgeons favor dorsal placement in both bulbar and urethral strictures, whereas others opt for ventral placement [26–31]. Although several studies have demonstrated comparable success rates for dorsal and ventral onlay grafting, the author of this chapter favors the use of dorsal placement of the graft in the penile urethra because the spongiosal vascularity in the ventral urethra is thinner and the graft support is less reliable when compared to the dorsal urethral surface.

Flaps: detailed knowledge of the blood supply to the penile skin and corpus spongiosum is mandatory for successful tissue harvest and transfer (see Section 2). Rather than rely on the recipient site for survival, flaps depend on their native blood supply containing pedicle for transfer. Flaps can be classified by their blood supply, harvest technique or their method of transfer. Several types of flaps have been used in urethral reconstruction: penile skin, hairless scrotal skin, gracilis muscle, and the forearm or upper arm as free flaps or (microvascular free-transfer flaps). Popularized in the past, scrotal skin flaps are random rotational flaps that can be used for urethral and genital reconstruction [32–36]. However, their use for urethral reconstruction was associated with unacceptable long-term complications. They were predominantly used for repair of complex bulbar urethral strictures as these flaps were difficult to reach the penile urethra because of their short pedicle. They are practically abandoned.

Various penile skin flaps have been described, which can be raised ventrally or dorsally on the penile shaft and taken longitudinally or circumferentially [37–39]. These flaps are fasciocutaneous in nature and are based on dartos fascia pedicle. The ventral, longitudinal flap, as described by Orandi, is best suited for penile shaft urethral strictures that do not reach the base of the penis or any part proximal to the penoscrotal angle because hair-bearing skin will inevitably be involved in the reconstruction. On the contrary, the transverse, circumferential preputial/distal penile skin flaps are long enough to bridge defects of the entire penile urethra and most of the bulbar urethra for example in panurethral defects. Ideally, flaps should be hairless, adapted to a moist environment, with a reliable vascular pedicle, mobile, and cosmetic. In general, anterior urethral reconstruction with the use of flaps has become less prevalent due to the increased popularity of oral mucosa grafts. A rise in prevalence of genital and urethral LS has also contributed to the near abdication of the use of flaps. Nonetheless, island skin flaps still find an important indication in reoperative cases with extensive spongiofibrosis and ischemic urethral mucosal plates where chances of graft take are minimal. These circumstances occur after irradiation, severe trauma, or infection.

One-stage vs. two (multiple)-stage reconstruction: in the past, most penile urethral strictures were repaired through a staged approach [40–43]. However, because of advancements with pediatric hypospadias surgery, adult noncomplicated penile urethral strictures are now more commonly repaired with single-stage procedures. In 1995, Bracka described a two-stage urethral reconstruction, which enables a versatile approach to surgical reconstruction of previously failed, complex penile urethral strictures, especially hypospadias cripples [42]. The Johanson marsupialization was developed and subsequently reserved for penile urethral strictures [43].

Repairs in adults who failed hypospadias repair in childhood pose a particular reconstructive challenge because of dense scarring, tissue inelasticity, inflammation, impaired blood supply, and penile and urethral shortening from previous, often multiple, operations [44–47]. Penile urethroplasty should be performed in a single stage, whenever feasible, to avoid discomfort and disability to the patient from a multistage repair. Most strictures associated with trauma, infection, or instrumentation, where the penile skin, dartos fascia and spongiosum are not significantly damaged, can be approached through a single-stage procedure. On the other hand, presence of local infection or inflammation associated with a specific underlying disease process obliterated urethral segments with dense surrounding fibrosis, and a history of prior interventions, especially prior flap or hypospadias repairs, are contraindications for single-stage repairs and, therefore, should not be advised. The two-stage reconstruction involves surgical opening of the stricture, augmentation, or substitution (more commonly with use of oral mucosa grafting) of the diseased urethral segment and creation of temporary urethrostomy for drainage (first stage), followed between 4 and 6 months later by neourethral tubularization (second stage). Therefore, it should be confined to situations where it is inappropriate to maintain the axial integrity of the urethral plate and a full circumference urethral reconstruction is mandatory.

7. Urethral reconstruction by stricture location

In order to facilitate description and discussion of the various surgical procedures used for adult penile urethral reconstruction, we will group them according to stricture location in the urethra: (1) external meatus and fossa navicularis and (2) penile shaft urethra. Furthermore, a separate section will be devoted to procedures used for previously failed repairs or reoperative procedures (**Table 2**).

7.1 External meatus and fossa navicularis

Strictures involving exclusively the external meatus may be treated with **dilatation** if the stricture is not obliterative or the scarred tissue is minimal, the urethral lumen is still patent and elastic. It is considered palliative and should be attempted only once. Strictures associated with LS rarely respond to conservative options, such as dilatation, urethrotomy, and meatotomy.

Meatotomy/meatoplasty: either ventral or dorsal, meatotomy can be used for select meatal strictures. A ventral or dorsal midline incision is performed sharply, and the resultant mucosal edges are everted and reapproximated to the glans using 4–0 or 5–0 absorbable sutures. The dorsal side should be avoided, which can bleed profusely by cutting into the highly vascularized spongiosal tissue of the glans. The ventral approach usually leaves the patient with a slight degree of hypospadias that is usually well tolerated. The goal is to create a patent 22–24 F urethral lumen, particularly in cases of LS. Adjuvant topical therapy may be helpful. Meatal strictures that need meatoplasty usually require concomitant reconstruction of the fossa navicularis.

In 2004, Malone described a technique to relieve stenosis of the external urinary meatus resulting from LS [48]. The procedure is rapid and easy to perform on an outpatient basis, providing good cosmesis and functional voiding without spraying. The meatotomy is carried out dorsally avoiding a hypospadiac meatus. If the stricture extends into the fossa navicularis, oral mucosa graft reconstruction is performed. The final result is a slit-shaped with good caliber meatus at the tip of the glans. The procedure has been successfully reproduced by others [49].

Longitudinal skin flap techniques: initially reported in the early 1960s, it is based on the Y-V principle and used for short strictures of the meatus and fossa navicularis [50, 51]. Good outcomes can be achieved with these techniques, especially in patients with strictures resulting from instrumentation such as a large bore catheter or transurethral resection and those that are not associated with LS. The use of genital skin in LS patients has a high failure rate.

Several variants have been reported. Cohney in 1963 described a penile flap procedure based on a circumferential elevated random penile skin flap. The distal urethra is well open, but the patient is left with a less appealing cosmetic result and a retrusive meatus (**Figure 7A** and **B**). Blandy-Tresidder in 1967 developed a flap procedure based on dartos fascia vascularity. It also provides good functional outcomes, but only modest improvement of the cosmetic final appearance. The meatus is usually left at the coronal level (**Figure 7C** and **D**). The Brannen flap repair [52], a modification of Blandy's procedure, was described in 1976 to try to create a better cosmetic appearance of the glans and distal penile segment [53]. However, some mechanical problems associated with the flap advancement make this procedure inefficient and, therefore, offer marginal improvement in terms of cosmesis (**Figure 7E** and **F**). Designed to create a cosmetically normal meatus and glans penis, De Sy in 1984 further modified the Blandy and Brannen techniques using an advancement midline skin island flap [54]. However, the proximal portion of the flap is de-epithelialized leaving a distal skin island on dartos fascia (**Figure 7G** and **H**). Again, the mechanics of the flap advancement is inefficient.

A. Ext. meatus and fossa navicularis

- Meatotomy/meatoplasty
- Longitudinal skin flap techniques
    - Cohney [50]
    - Blandy-Tresidder [51]
    - Brannen [52]
    - De Sy [53]
- Transverse ventral/circumferential fasciocutaneous skin island flaps
    - Jordan [54]
    - McAninch [39]
- Graft techniques
    - Tubularized full-thickness skin graft (Devine, 1979)
    - Inner prepuce [41]
    - OMG [41]
- Combination of grafts and flaps [65]
- Endourethroplasty techniques
    - Nandé (1998)
    - Nikolavsky et al. [64]
- Staged techniques
    - Bracka [41]
    - Jordan (2009)
- Tubularized incised plate urethroplasty
    - Snodgrass [58]

B. Penile shaft urethra

- Flap reconstruction
    - Orandi flap [37]
    - Quartey flap [67]
    - Mcflinch flap (1993)
    - Turner-Warwick flap (1993)
- Graf reconstructions
    - Dorsal OMG onlay (Barbagli, 1996)
    - Dorsal OMG inlay by ventral urethrotomy [59]
    - Penile inversion and one-sided dorsolateral OMG graft tech [75]
- Staged reconstructions
    - Johanson's techniques [40]
    - Mesh graft urethroplasty [77]
    - Staged OMG urethroplasty
- Tissue engineering/stem cell therapy

Table 2.
Urethral reconstruction by stricture location.

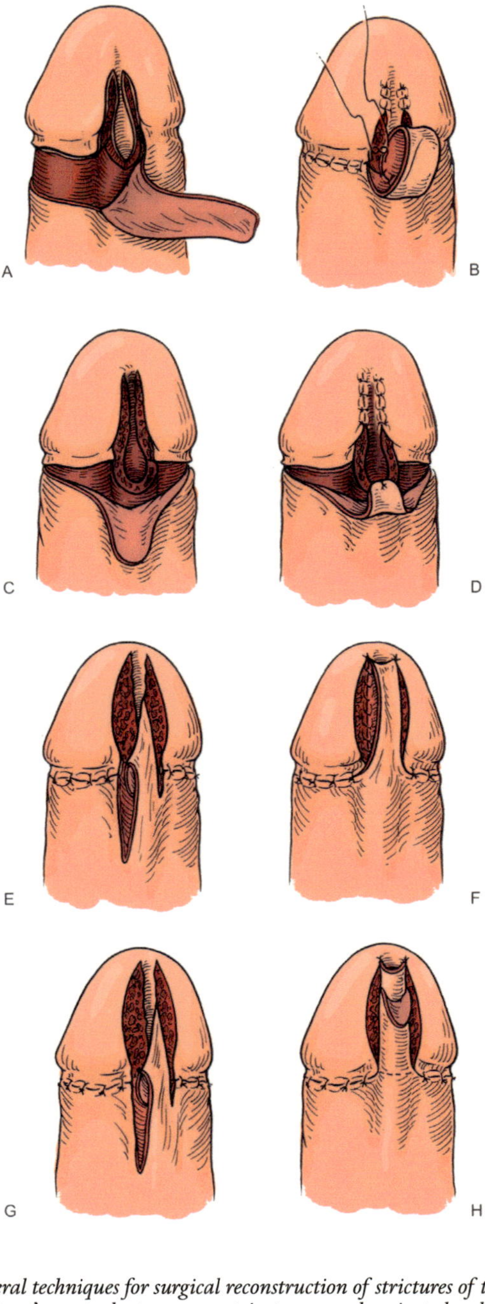

Figure 7.
Schematic illustration of several techniques for surgical reconstruction of strictures of the urethral meatus and fossa navicularis. (A, B) Cohney's meatoplasty: an eccentric, transversely oriented, subcoronal flap is developed, and the urethrotomy is extended to normal urethra. The transverse flap is rotated into the urethrotomy defect. (C, D) Blandy's meatoplasty: creation of a midline flap. Urethrotomy is extended till normal urethral lumen. The flap is advanced into the urethrotomy defect. (E, F) Brannen's meatoplasty: a longer midline dartos-based flap is developed and is then widely advanced. (G, H) De Sy's meatoplasty: a midline flap similar to Brannen' technique is mobilized. The proximal portion of the flap is de-epithelialized leaving a distal skin island attached to a dartos pedicle. The de-epithelialized surface of the flap is anastomosed, and the ventral glans is reapproximated over the reconstruction (from Jordan and McCammon [96]).

Transverse ventral fasciocutaneous skin island flap: as initially described by Jordan, this is a broad-based penile skin island flap oriented transversally on the ventral penile skin and elevated on a dartos fascia pedicle [55]. Minimal flap advancement is required, and the cosmetic appearance is virtually normal (**Figure 8**). McAninch modified this technique avoiding any disruption of the ventral glanular

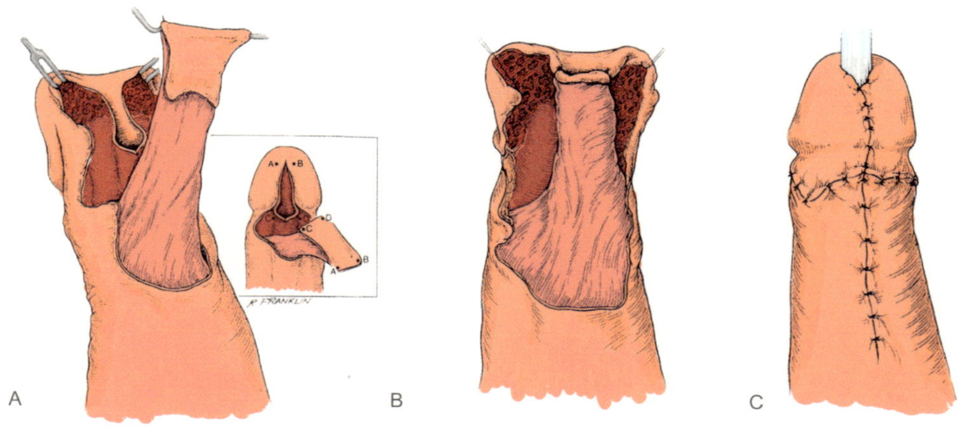

Figure 8.
Schematic illustration of Jordan's ventral transverse skin island flap procedure. (A–C) After urethrotomy is made till normal urethra, a ventral skin island flap is elevated above Buck's fascia, and the lateral glans wings are exposed. The skin island is rotated, transposed, and inverted into the urethrotomy defect. The glans wings are sutured ventrally. Inset shows details of the rotation, transposition, and inversion of the flap (from Jordan and McCammon [96]).

integrity, which he assumed to provide a superior cosmetic result. This would be of paramount importance to the patient, overshadowing the functional success of the reconstruction. In his technique, the glans is exposed in either a glans-cap or a glans-wings fashion (**Figure 9**) [56, 57].

Graft techniques: penile skin grafts were first employed and preferred tissue for urethroplasty before the advent of oral mucosa. Devine described a procedure using a tubularized full-thickness skin graft to reconstruct the external meatus and fossa navicularis [58]. Bracka reported in 2008 that the inner prepuce can be used for postischemic or infectious scarring as it is thin, flexible, with a reliable take, adapted to a moist environment and with no potential for hair growth (**Figure 10**) [43]. If not available, then postauricular skin graft is an acceptable alternative if oral mucosa cannot be harvested. However, due to its physical and biological characteristics, abundance, easy harvesting with minimal impact on the concealed donor site, and low oral morbidity, oral mucosa has become the most popular material for substitution or augmentation in urethral stricture repair. Oral mucosa can be used in strictures related to LS. It can be used in a single or staged procedure. Single-stage procedures are appropriate if the urethral plate is salvageable. In 1994, Snodgrass described a technique for the correction of pediatric hypospadias, which involved incision of the urethral plate followed by tubularization and secondary healing of the incised plate [59]. Although it produces good results in children, this procedure has not been associated with similar results in adults, often requiring inlay OMGs to increase the urethral lumen diameter [60]. Endourethroplasty techniques emerged in the early 1980s [61]. A few variants were reported later [62, 63]. However, due to inherent technical difficulties and complications of surgical reconstruction of distal penile and fossa navicularis strictures, these procedures have not become popular. Recently, Nikolavsky et al. has introduced a novel surgical technique for the reconstruction of distal urethral strictures using OMG through a transurethral approach with encouraging initial results (**Figures 11** and **12**) [64]. They designed this novel and elegant surgical concept in order to avoid the complications, technical difficulties, and limitations of the previous procedures used in this urethral area. The surgical procedure is applicable to the entire distal penile urethra, avoids an external ventral skin incision, preserves the glans penis, and employs oral mucosa for grafting, thus

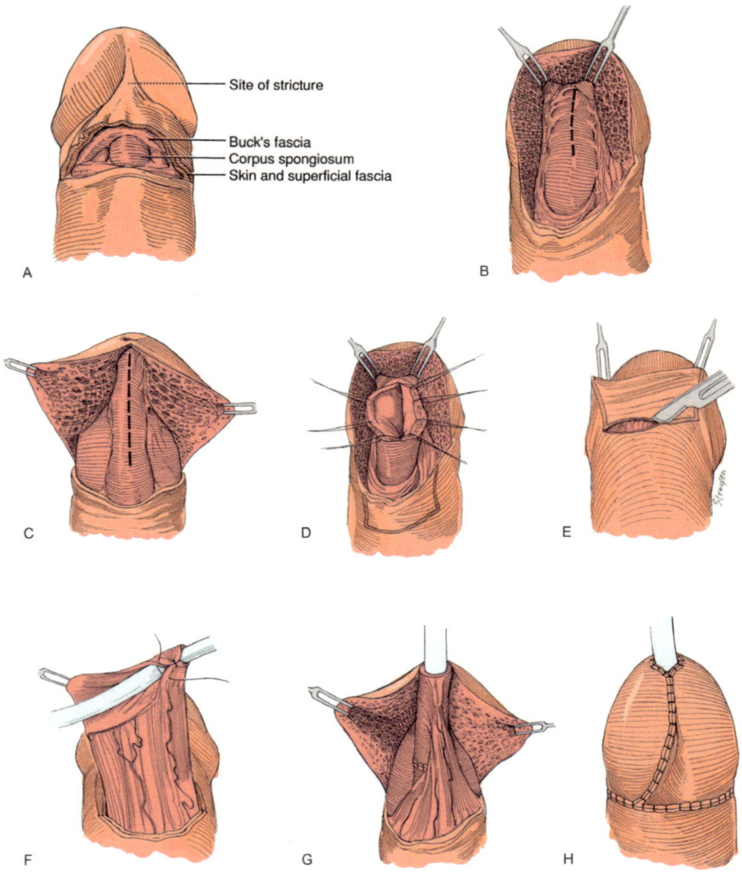

Figure 9.
Fasciocutaneous distal penile flap urethroplasty as described by McAninch. (A–H) Urethral exposure followed by ventral longitudinal urethrotomy. The fossa navicularis is exposed with either a glans-cap or a glans-wings technique. A fasciocutaneous distal, transverse, ventral penile flap is developed. The urethral stricture can be corrected by either a ventral onlay or a neourethral tube. The glans wings or cap is sutured to cover the flap reconstruction (from Armenakas and McAninch [97]).

achieving both excellent functional and cosmetic results. This procedure is especially indicated for patients affected by LS-related distal strictures, where only oral mucosal grafts are advised.

Combined flap and graft technique: in 2011, Gelman and Sohn described a procedure combining a dorsal onlay graft with a ventral onlay flap for a subset of patient with ischemic, obliterated distal strictures who had already failed urethral repair, or who had a history of hypospadias [65]. This procedure is particularly useful in strictures associated with compromised urethral plates due to ischemia and dense scarring from previous repairs and when a two-stage procedure is not desired (**Figure 13**).

Staged techniques: these techniques are best suited for patients who have failed hypospadias repairs or the urethral plate is deficient or densely scarred, or if there is involvement of LS. These techniques may be considered more versatile than flap repairs and are preferred in patients with LS. The modern staged urethral reconstruction described by Bracka in 1995 is a versatile approach to difficult anterior urethral reconstructions [41–43]. In Bracka's procedure, the diseased urethra is excised entirely and the urethral plate is replaced by an OM onlay graft (**Figure 10**). Jordan later described a similar technique [66].

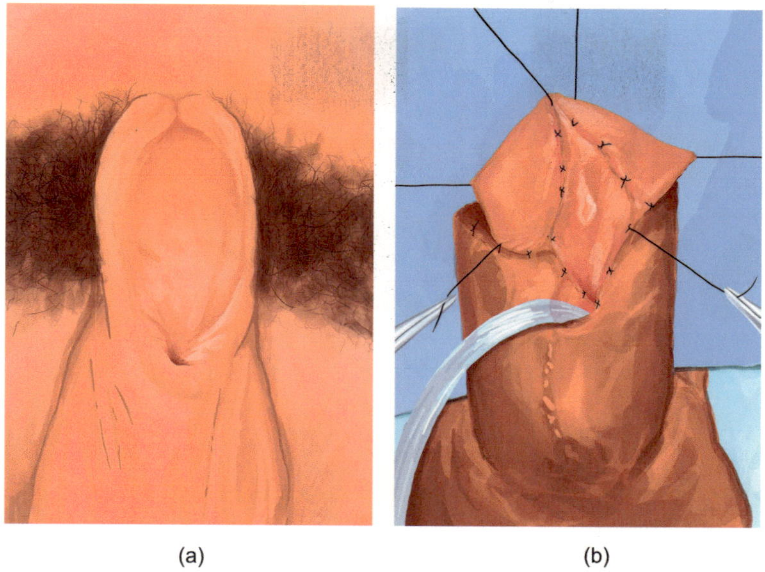

Figure 10.
Two-stage distal urethra reconstruction as described by Bracka. (a–b) Marsupialization of the urethra and placement of the oral mucosal graft after excision of the diseased urethral mucosa at the first stage. Aspect of the graft 6 months later, which is then prepared for tubularization at the second stage.

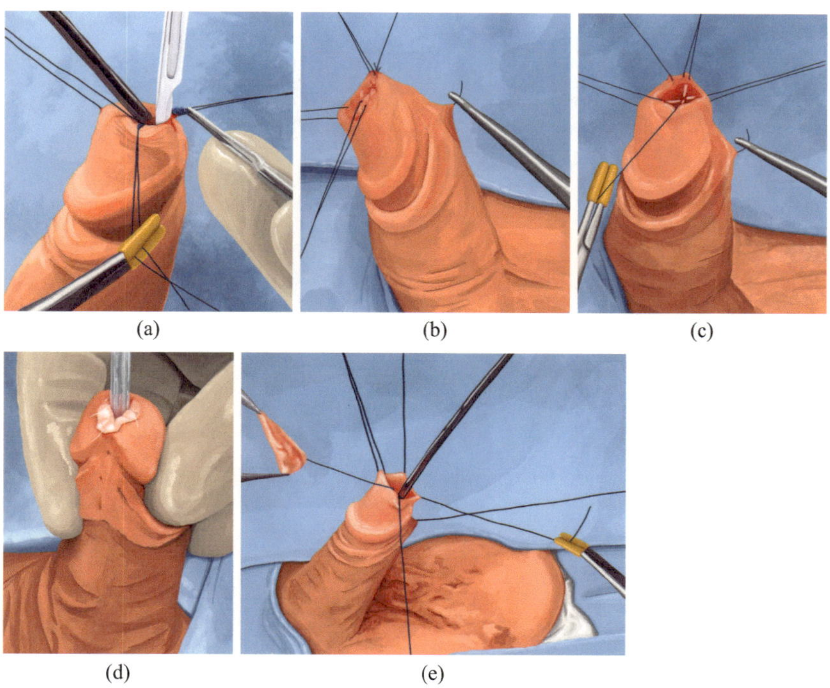

Figure 11.
Transurethral ventral buccal mucosa graft inlay urethroplasty for reconstruction of fossa navicularis and distal urethral meatus as described by Nikolavsky. (a-e) Transurethral ventral shallow resection of scar tissue. Placement of double-armed suture through buccal graft and through apex of urethrotomy (inside out). External apical suture tying, meatal BMG edge fixation, and additional inside-out quilting of the graft with double-armed sutures (reproduced with permission from Springer Science + Business Media Dordrecht, Ref. [62]).

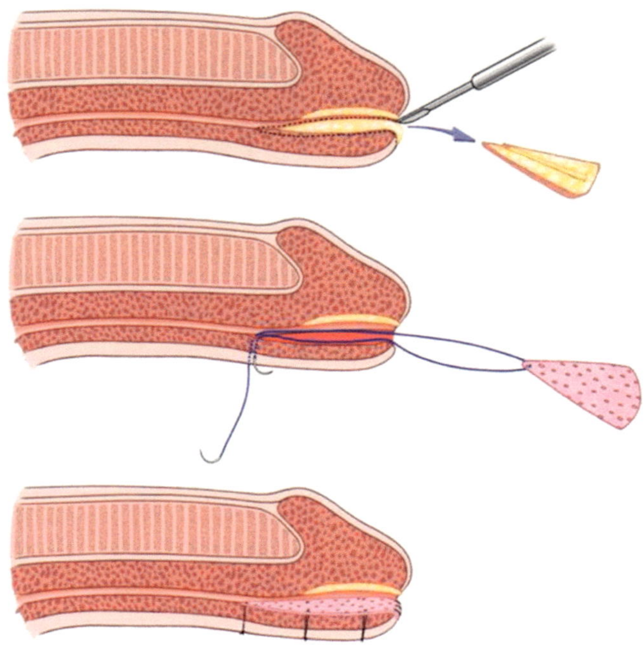

Figure 12.
Intraoperative demonstration of the procedure described in ***Figure 11*** *(reproduced with permission from Springer Science + Business Media Dordrecht, Ref. [62]).*

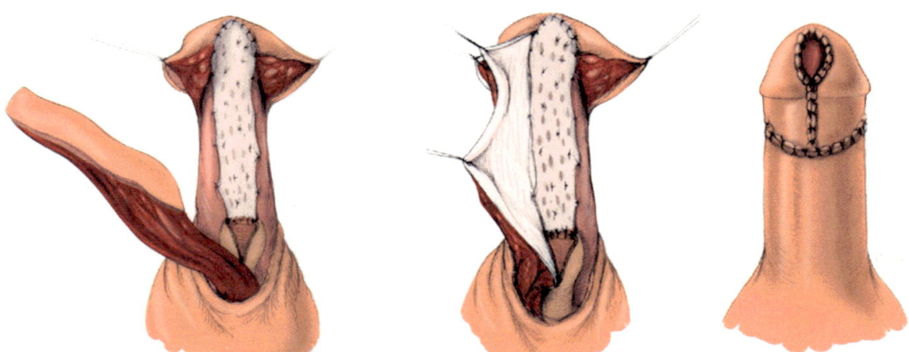

Figure 13.
Schematic illustration of single-stage, combined flap graft technique as described by Gelman. (A–C) Oral mucosal graft is placed and quilted dorsally followed by closure of the urethrotomy defect by a penile skin flap (from Gelman and Sohn, Ref. [63]).

7.2 Penile shaft urethra

For penile shaft urethral strictures, a stricturotomy and onlay or inlay patch graft, or alternatively a flap reconstruction, can be used for simple strictures. More complex cases may eventually require total excision of the strictured area and circumferential reconstruction with OM grafts or penile skin flap. In more complex situations, such as after previous failed repairs and compromised or obliterated urethras, a staged reconstruction is preferable. Penile urethral strictures are rarely cured by dilatation or DVIU. If either of these procedures fail once, the chance of a better outcome with a second attempt is almost nil, making urethroplasty the only curative option. Anastomotic urethroplasty should be avoided in the penile urethra, even in short strictures, as ventral curvature usually occurs.

Patient advanced age and comorbidities may steer the urologist away from open surgery. In these circumstances, periodic urethral (self)-dilatation or definitive urethrostomy should be strongly considered.

Flap reconstructions: penile skin island flaps may be elevated in a longitudinal or transverse, circumferential fashion, and variants.

Orandi flap: the Orandi flap is a longitudinal, ventral, fasciocutaneous island penile flap that is appropriate for single-stage reconstruction of strictures of the penile shaft urethra [37]. Inclusion of the distal bulbar urethra in the reconstruction may be hampered by hair-bearing skin of the more proximal part of the flap. Careful planning of the flap is critical before skin incision to avoid jeopardizing the flap design and its blood supply. The flap must be handled meticulously with the use of atraumatic surgical tools and eventually loupe magnification. It then must be mobilized gently to preserve its arterial and venous blood supply. The type and size of suture material is paramount to minimize tissue reaction.

With the penis on stretch, a longitudinal nonhair-bearing skin island is marked on the ventral aspect of the penis. The description of the surgical technique is outlined in **Figure 14**. The penis is snugly dressed to avoid hematoma. Drains are rarely required. Patients are kept on strict bed rest for 3–5 days to minimize swelling. Intravenous antibiotics are administered for at least 48 h, followed by oral antibiotic prophylaxis for one additional week. Erections should be avoided. The use of a suprapubic catheter for urinary drainage is not mandatory but preferable, which should be kept for 2 weeks. The urethral catheter is left plugged to act as a stent only. After 2–3 weeks, the urethral catheter is removed and the patient is sent home with the suprapubic tube occluded, allowing the patient to resume urethral voiding. The suprapubic tube is removed after a few days of normal urethral voiding. If a

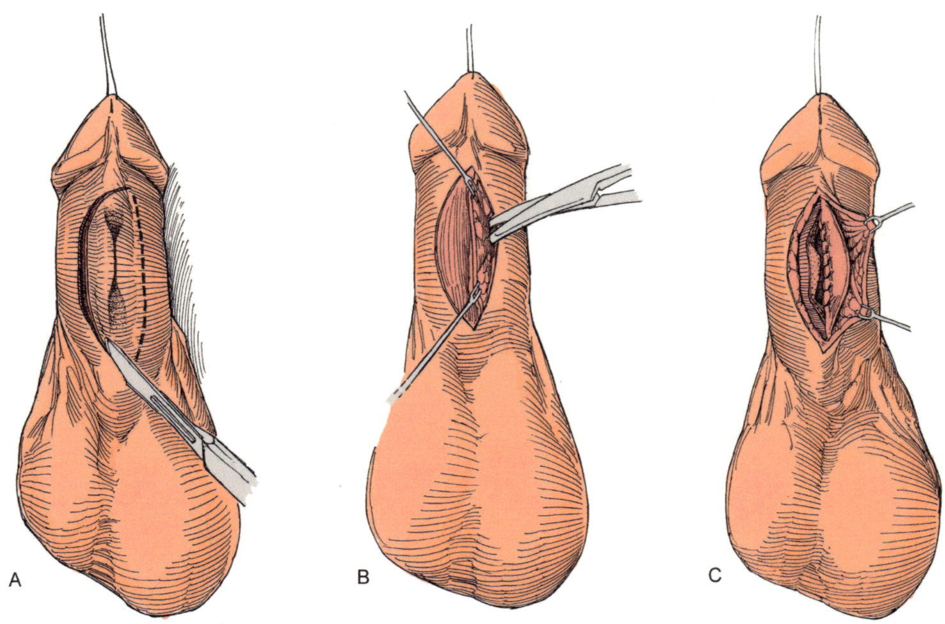

Figure 14.
Orandi flap procedure. (A–C) Deep skin incision is made over the strictured urethra. Dotted line indicates skin incision. Dartos pedicled flap is created lateral to the superficial skin incision, which will cover the urethrotomy defect. The skin is closed in the midline (from Elliott and McAninch [98]).

fistula develops, the urethral catheter is not reinserted and the suprapubic diversion is maintained for another week. If still persistent, then it should be repaired after 4–6 months.

The Orandi flap is a reliable and relatively easy flap to harvest. It is a useful solution for a single-stage reconstruction of penile urethral strictures.

Quartey flap: in 1983, Quartey described a one-stage flap urethroplasty technique using a transverse distal penile or preputial island of skin as a flap, which is supplied axially by the superficial external pudendal vessels for penile urethral strictures with possible extended application to the entire penile and bulbar urethra and even difficult posterior urethral strictures [67, 68]. He described the possibility of this island of skin being used either as a patch or as a tube. In very long strictures, the complete circumference of the distal penile skin can be extended ventrally and proximally toward the base of the penis in the hairless area. This flap design granted it the term "hockey stick island flap" (**Figure 15**).

McAninch flap: in 1993, McAninch reported the initial circular fasciocutaneous penile skin flap for the reconstruction of extensive anterior urethral strictures [39]. This flap is a variant of the flap described by Quartey 10 years earlier with the difference that this fasciocutaneous flap uses Buck's fascia as a paddle to carry the vascular pedicle to the distal flap skin. It can provide a hairless flap up to 15 cm in length, making this flap, like Quartey's flap, extremely versatile. It can be used in uncircumcised as well as circumcised men. The width of the flap varies from 2.0 to 2.5 cm, depending on the stricture characteristics. With the penis on traction, the distal incision is

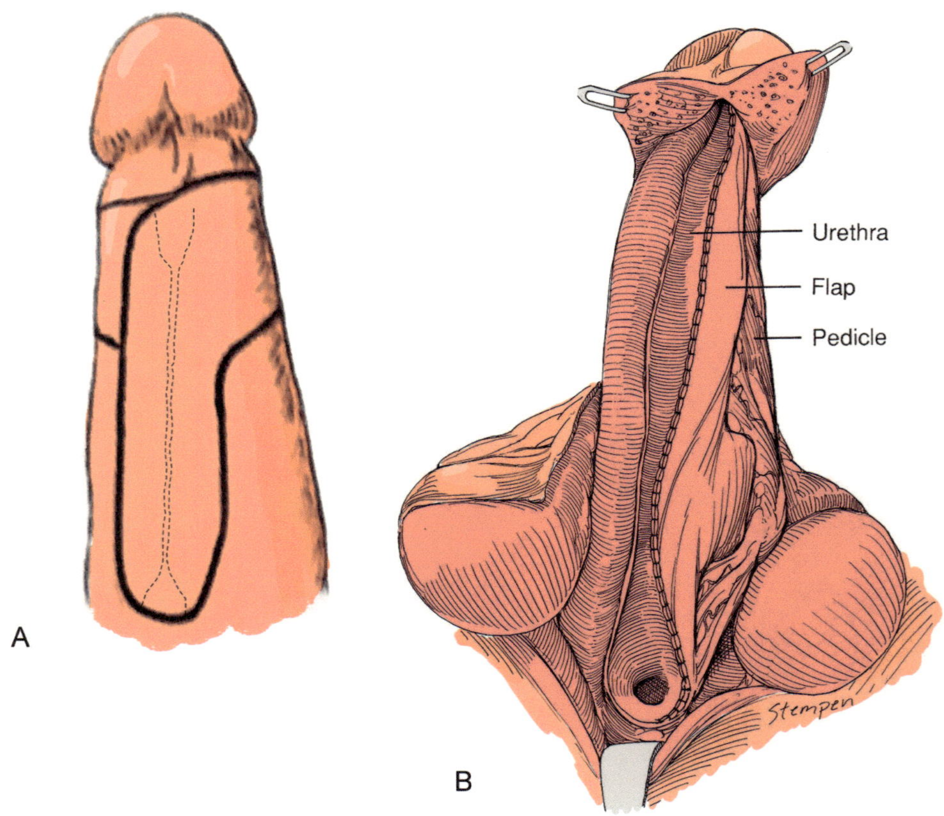

Figure 15.
Quartey flap procedure. (A, B) Hockey stick skin island flap is fashioned. The length of the flap may be tailored as needed. After ventral longitudinal urethrotomy, the flap is anastomosed similar to the Orandi technique.

carried down deeply beneath the pedicle just beneath Buck's fascia, but superficial to the dorsal neurovascular bundle (dorsally), circumflex vessels (laterally), and urethra (ventrally). The proximal incision extends proximally to the base of the penis through a dissection plane beneath the skin and subdermal or dartos fascia (**Figure 16**). The flap and pedicle can be divided either ventrally or dorsally and rotated to cover the urethral area as an onlay flap. This flap also allows reconstruction of complex strictures of various lengths in a single stage even in circumcised patients. The cosmetic and functional results are excellent in experienced hands.

Turner-Warwick flap: described by Turner-Warwick, this is a bilateral, longitudinal, ventral-based pedicle skin flap supported by right and left ventrolateral branches of the external pudendal artery. Although it may be employed in penile urethral stricture repair, this flap is most useful in bulbar urethral reconstruction [69].

Graft reconstructions: historically, grafts have been used for reconstruction of anterior urethral strictures since the early 1960s [70]. Several different types of graft material have been used with favorable results since then, but in the modern era, oral mucosa has become the graft of choice for its excellent graft characteristics and ease and low morbidity of harvest.

Dorsal OMG onlay technique (Barbagli): ventral onlay grafts are usually discouraged on the corpus spongiosum if the penile urethra is thin, not allowing spongioplasty maneuvers to support the graft and optimize graft take. Therefore, a dorsal onlay approach is used in this urethral segment. The urethra can be exposed either through a circular, subcoronal incision followed by penile shaft degloving, or a ventral midline incision, the latter one being favored by the author of this chapter for its associated lower local morbidity. After identifying the obstruction of a soft 20F Nelaton catheter or Bougie-a-Boule, the urethra is mobilized circumferentially off of the corpora cavernosa along the stricture length. The urethra is rotated 180° for preparation of the dorsal urethrotomy after placing marking stitches at both ends of the stricture. The graft is quilted to the corpora cavernosa, and the edges of the graft and urethrotomy are sewn together. Barbagli et al. have suggested the use of fibrin glue for one-stage penile graft urethroplasty. The authors reported that this new adjunct was safe and effective, with limited complications and satisfactory preliminary outcomes [71].

Dorsal OMG inlay through a ventral sagittal urethrotomy (Asopa): in 2001, Asopa described the technique of dorsal OMG inlay through a ventral sagittal urethrotomy approach as an alternative to the Barbagli technique for the repair of penile strictures (**Figure 17**). The advantages are a simpler dissection, no mobilization of the urethra, and preservation of the urethral blood supply through circumflex and

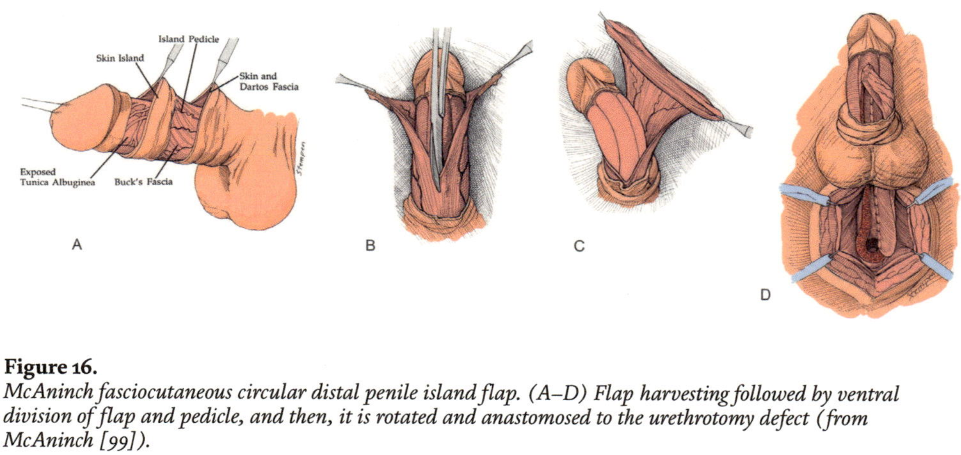

Figure 16.
McAninch fasciocutaneous circular distal penile island flap. (A–D) Flap harvesting followed by ventral division of flap and pedicle, and then, it is rotated and anastomosed to the urethrotomy defect (from McAninch [99]).

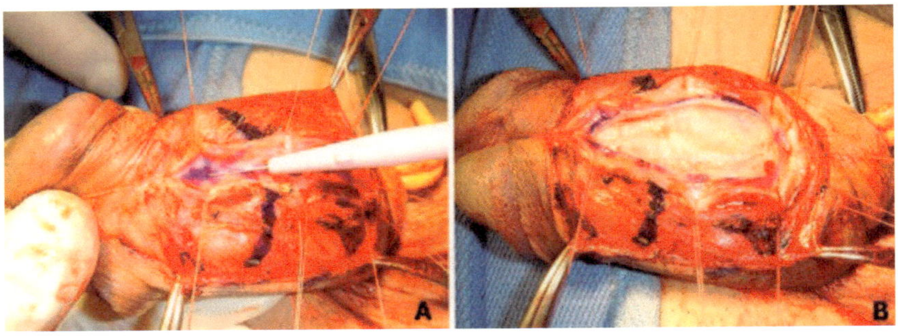

Figure 17.
(A-B) Asopa technique used in long penile urethral stricture approached through a ventral incision.

perforating vessels [72]. However, it involves an extra urethrotomy, which may potentially lead to additional urethral trauma. In the bulbar urethra, it can be used in combination with a second ventrally placed graft. Again, either a degloving or a ventral midline incision can be used. An alternative perineal approach for exclusive penile urethral strictures has been recently adapted from the Kulkarni perineal approach to panurethral stricture repair (**Figure 18**) [73, 74]. This perineal approach avoids the morbidity and less optimal cosmetic results of a penile incision and scar, allowing the performance of penile graft urethroplasty through either Barbagli's dorsal onlay or Asopa's dorsal inlay or Kulkarni's one-sided dorsolateral approach with equivalent functional results.

Penile inversion and one-sided dorsolateral OMG graft technique (*Kulkarni*): Kulkarni first described the technique of perineal approach with penile inversion to expose the full length of anterior urethra for reconstruction of panurethral strictures with avoidance of a penile incision. In 2009, he reported and popularized a slight but important modification of his original technique, which involved a one-sided urethral dissection [75]. The preservation of the one-sided vascular supply to the urethra and its entire muscular and neurogenic support should represent a slight but significant step toward perfecting the surgical technique of urethral reconstruction using a minimally invasive approach. The preservation of the vascular blood supply

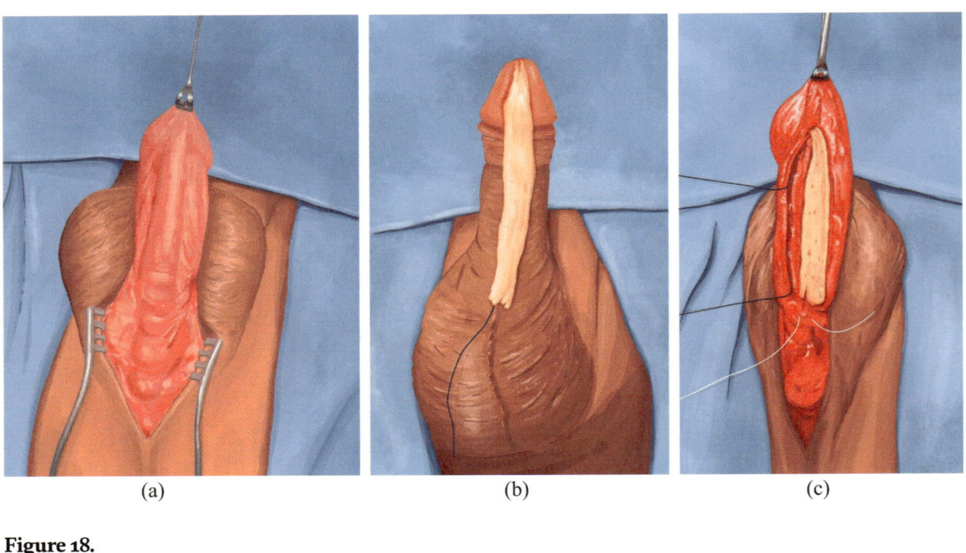

Figure 18.
Kulkarni's one-sided dorsal onlay graft for anterior urethroplasty for long urethral strictures. (a-c) The penile shaft has been inverted into the perineum where the entire reconstruction is performed. This technique can be used to repair the entire length of the anterior urethra (reproduced with permission from Sanjay Kulkarni, MD).

to one side of the urethra along with its muscular and neural support had a significant impact on functional outcomes. The whole operation is performed through the perineal approach only, making this a minimally invasive approach (**Figure 18**).

Staged reconstructions: staged urethroplasty is used for complicated strictures with significant scar tissue involved, failed hypospadias repair, multiple prior urethroplasty failures, long obliterative strictures, presence of diverticulum or fistulation, and strictures caused by lichen sclerosus, where complete removal of the native diseased urethra may be necessary. In all these circumstances, there is absence of enough healthy tissue to allow a successful one-stage reconstruction. Staged reconstructions are based on the marsupialization of the strictured urethra and involve a planned repair strategy characterized by more than one operation and inherent free tissue transfer. Classically, the term "two-stage urethroplasty" is a misnomer as a significant number of these patients end up requiring more than two operations to produce the final result, that is, a patent tubularized urethra [76]. Alternatives to staged urethroplasty are definitive perineal urethrostomy, combined double face grafting, or other less common individualized procedures.

Johanson's technique: in the first stage, the penis is placed on stretch and the distal end of the stricture is identified. A longitudinal penile skin incision is carried out over the strictured area. The stricturotomy is extended proximally until normal urethra is exposed. The lateral edges of the urethra are sewn with the skin edges (**Figure 19**). Because voiding in a standing position is not possible without dribbling, soiling of the scrotum, and a forward stream, patients may be offered a temporary perineal urethrostomy, if necessary, which is closed at the second stage of the reconstruction. At the second stage, the urethral plate is tubularized and a dartos flap is developed to cover the suture line to avoid fistulation.

Mesh graft urethroplasty: this procedure was first described by Schreiter and Noll [77]. In the first stage, a longitudinal incision is made over the strictured urethra. The urethra is marsupialized preserving the native urethral plate. The split thickness graft (or foreskin) is harvested in the standard fashion with an

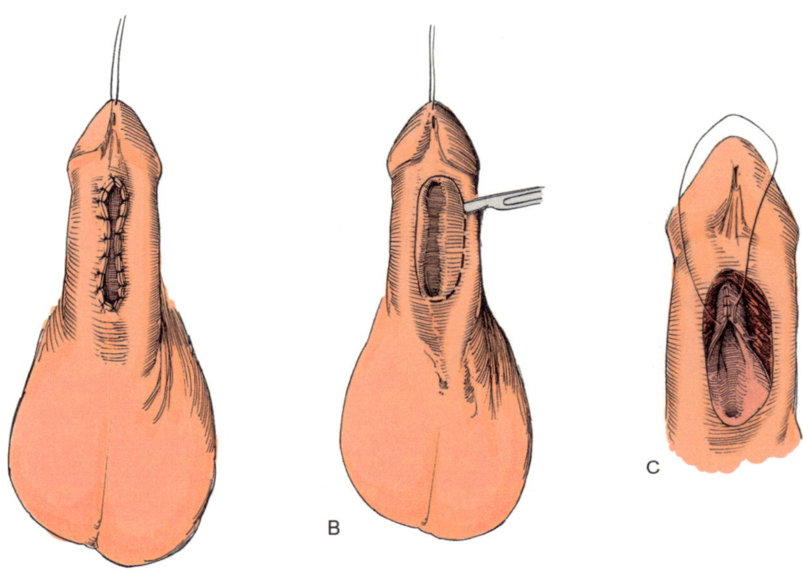

Figure 19.
Johanson's two-stage procedure. (A–C) The anastomosis of the skin edges and the longitudinal urethrotomy is performed at the first stage. The urethrotomy is fashioned as a neourethral tube at the second stage. Modification with use of oral mucosal graft has been described.

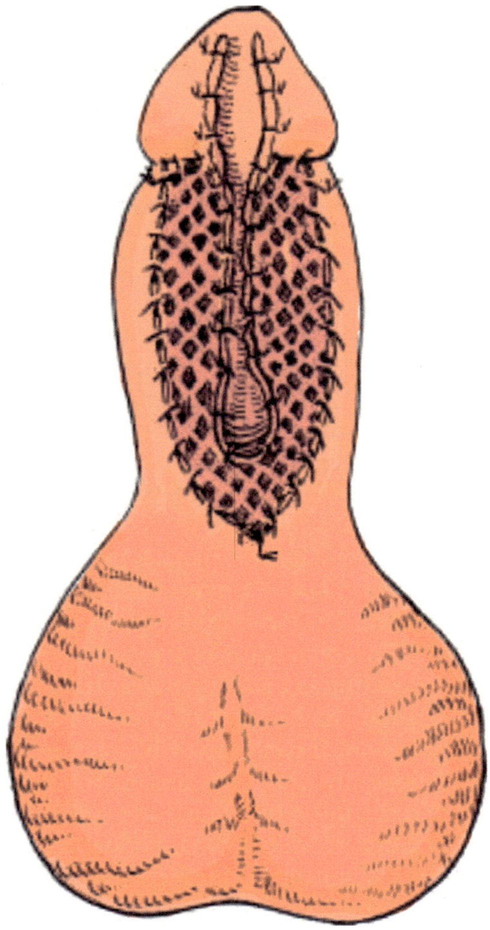

Figure 20.
Mesh graft urethroplasty as described by Schreiter. Meshed skin graft has been placed on the wound ground and quilted to the host bed (first stage). The prepared urethral plate is tubularized approximately 6 months later (second stage).

electrical dermatome and is meshed with a mechanical skin mesher using a 1:15 ratio sheet. The graft is placed on the wound ground lateral to the preserved urethral plate (**Figure 20**). The graft is fixed by running 5–0 monofilament sutures. The second stage (urethral tubularization) is performed in a standard fashion. In a study by Carr et al., success was achieved in 80% at a median follow-up of 38 months [78].

Staged oral mucosa graft urethroplasty: today, staged reconstructions using oral mucosal grafts has become a reliable and the most popular procedure to treat difficult anterior urethral strictures that are not amenable to single-stage graft or flap reconstructions. The indications are similar to the procedures described above. The surgical technique is generally similar (to variants) and based on the technique used for the Johanson and Schreiter's operations, that is, urethral marsupialization in the first stage followed by urethral tubularization 4–6 months later, the OMG being placed at the first stage. At times, it may be necessary to use additional grafts at the time of tubularization to optimize the urethral plate. This is the procedure of choice for strictures associated with LS. Success rates are very good when compared to earlier techniques with an acceptable number of surgical revisions. Multistage urethroplasty should replace "two-stage" urethroplasty as the accepted terminology as it is not uncommon for patients to require more than two procedures to complete successful tubularization. This may lead to more realistic patient expectations as well. Although completion of the second stage may not always be necessary for functional improvement, cosmetic outcomes with restoration of a glanular meatus can be excellent and achieved in the majority of patients [79]. An algorithm of surgical reconstruction of strictures of the meatus, fossa navicularis, and penile urethral shaft is suggested (**Figure 21**).

Tissue engineering, stem cell, and future: the field of tissue engineering and scar modulation is an exciting area of research in reconstructive urology and is rapidly progressing. Much research has been devoted to the development of a tissue-engineered urethral graft. Currently used grafts, when long, can cause initial donor site morbidity or may be insufficient. Researchers have investigated cell-free and cell-seeded grafts as substitutes for human urethra. There are different approaches to developing these grafts with variable reported successes in studies conducted in animal and human models. Further research may improve the management of long and complex urethral strictures that usually require oral mucosa substitution of urethroplasty with tissue-engineered grafts. These grafts have become necessary because the use of oral mucosa may be limited by its availability. A combination of buccal (cheek), lingual (tongue), and labial (lip) mucosa may be utilized and necessary in some cases. Patients with reduced mouth opening or previous oral surgery may have less oral tissue for use. In addition, longer grafts carry a greater morbidity. The risk of donor site morbidity is increased in smokers, tobacco chewers, and those with poor oral hygiene, which will contraindicate the use of oral mucosa, and, therefore, necessitate a tissue-engineered graft [80].

To generate new tissues, biomedical engineering investigators have utilized three basic tools: cells, scaffold, and growth factor. The earliest use of human cells dates back to approximately 30 years ago [81]. Several different tissue-engineered grafts have been used for urethral reconstruction. There are two types of urethral grafts: (1) those that contain living autologous cells and (2) those that are cell free. The latter include grafts obtained from cadaveric or animal sources. This tissue undergoes treatment to become completely cell free. The resultant biological

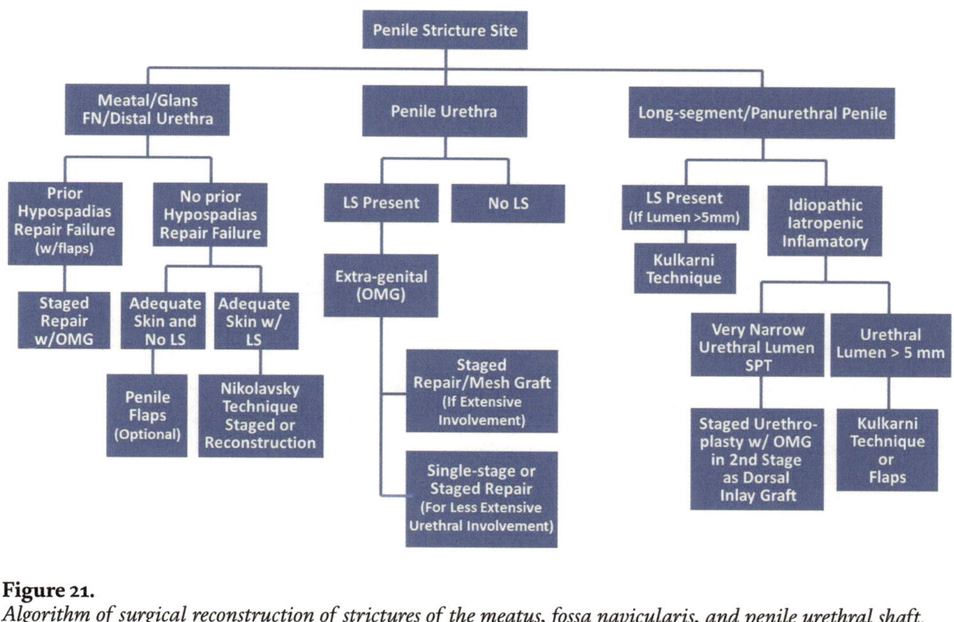

Figure 21.
Algorithm of surgical reconstruction of strictures of the meatus, fossa navicularis, and penile urethral shaft. FN = fossa navicularis, LS = lichen sclerosus, TIP = tubularized incised plate, and OMG = oral mucosal graft.

matrix is then implanted. A good vascular bed is needed to allow take and infiltration of host cells. As a rule, these techniques would only be expected to be particularly successful for substituting short urethral defects. In contrast, cellularized grafts contain a matrix populated with autologous cells, which are obtained from a small biopsy from the patient. The cells are cultured, expanded, and seeded onto the matrix. The matrix containing cells is then implanted onto the host bed [82].

A critical element required for successful tissue engineering is the cell source. Cells can be isolated from autologous urine-derived stems cells, smooth muscle cells, adipogenic, chondrogenic, and neural lineages [83]. Because simple cell injection to a target site is rarely feasible, a scaffold, or a template, also called artificial extracellular matrix, is necessary. The major function of a scaffold is to assist proliferation, differentiation, and biosynthesis of cells [84, 85].

Scar modulation represents another potential development that may revolutionize urethral reconstruction. Antifibrotic injectables, acting as scar inhibitors, may be placed into the stricture after stricturotomy. Stents impregnated with tacrolimus or paclitaxel have been tried in animal and human models with apparently promising early results [86, 87].

Regenerative medicine (cell therapy and tissue engineering) has made solid progress over the last three decades. We cautiously hope that these technologies will finally enter the routine clinical environment and be applicable in the treatment of urethral strictures/stenosis.

Sexual impact of anterior urethroplasty: overall, anterior urethroplasty appears to have minimal or no impact on long-term sexual dysfunction. One study revealed a moderate effect on sexual function, especially transient chordee in 25% of patients [88]. In another study, the impact of urethroplasty was not worse than circumcision [89]. Another study found a minimal impact on ejaculatory function [90]. One further study reported erectile dysfunction (ED) in approximately 40% of patients, although recovery occurred in most by 6 months. In this study, bulbar urethroplasty affected erectile function more than penile urethroplasty, probably explained by the proximity of the bulbar urethra to the erectile nerves [89]. Even staged urethroplasty does not seem to influence sexual function in patients undergoing penile urethroplasty, although many may experience *de novo* penile curvature, reduced penile length, and/or reduced penile sensitivity [91]. In conclusion, a meta-analysis conducted by Blaschko et al. found that the risk of *de novo* ED after anterior urethroplasty was low at 1% with most of the cases of the *de novo* ED resolving within 6–12 months; however, the possibility of *de novo* posturethroplasty ED, even if transient from the psychological impact of surgery or during revascularization, should be discussed during preoperative evaluation [92].

8. Lower urinary tract symptoms (LUTS) and urethral strictures

The spectrum of lower urinary tract symptoms (LUTS) at initial presentation for urethral stricture disease (USD) is well described. Anterior urethral stricture disease most commonly presents as urinary obstruction and may occasionally present as acute urinary retention. However, there is little data addressing these symptoms in patients after urethroplasty. LUTS after urethroplasty for anterior USD and the relationship of these symptoms to USD recurrence has also been observed [93]. It was reported that men with a successful outcome after urethroplasty tend to remain asymptomatic, whereas those who recur have LUTS, typically with weak urinary flow but without dysuria and hematuria. The authors supported the need for a USD-specific validated questionnaire to be used for follow-up after urethroplasty.

All men being evaluated for lower urinary tract symptoms (LUTS) should include urethral stricture in the differential diagnosis and include a combination of patient-reported symptom measures, uroflowmetry to assess severity of obstruction, and postvoid residual volume by ultrasound to determine degree of urinary retention. Patients with urethral stricture typically present a weak flow rate. However, evaluation of urethral stricture requires further specific testing to delineate the location, length of the stricture, and degree of narrowing such as urethroscopy and retrograde urethrogram with or without voiding cystourethrogram. LUTS are the usual clinical manifestation of urethral strictures, regardless of location, etiology, and severity. However, LUTS after urethral stricture repair are not uncommon. Urgency has been reported in 40% of men and urge incontinence in 12% of men after anterior urethroplasty. De novo urgency and urge incontinence is seen in 9 and 5% of men, respectively, after urethroplasty. Once a complication of urethroplasty (such as recurrent urethral stricture or diverticulum) has been excluded as a cause, evaluation of LUTS in such patients should focus on the differential diagnosis between bladder dysfunction (overactive bladder and underactive bladder) and other outlet obstructions (such as benign prostatic obstruction), dysfunctional voiding, or medical causes (such as nocturnal polyuria). Management of overactive bladder has different treatment options, which may include behavioral modification, physical therapy, anticholinergic, and/or beta-3 agonist medications. In more severe cases, intravesical onabotulinum toxin, sacral neuromodulation, or peripheral tibial nerve stimulation may be indicated. Definitive treatment for underactive bladder is limited in number and success. Although management of LUTS for patients after urethral stricture repair can usually proceed similarly as for patients without prior history of urethral reconstruction, special consideration and alterations in management need to be made when instrumenting the urethra, as the urethral lumen may be narrower in these patients.

Recently, an analysis of risk factors leading to postoperative urethral stricture and bladder neck contracture (BNC) following transurethral resection of prostate (TURP) has been performed [94]. The authors have found that lower resection speed, intraoperative urethral mucosal rupture, and postoperative continuous infection were associated with a higher risk of urethral stricture, whereas more severe storage symptoms and smaller prostate volumes were associated with a higher risk of BNC after TURP.

9. Future directions and goals

Penile urethroplasty has evolved significantly over the last eight decades, since the first attempts at reconstruction using preputial tubes or a staged approach using penile skin [95]. An improved understanding of the pathophysiology of LS and a high complication rate following skin-based reconstructions favored a shift to the use of oral mucosal grafts, particularly in LS strictures. To date, very little advances have been achieved with conservative/pharmacological therapeutic options to stabilize or modulate the scarring process of this recalcitrant cutaneous disease.

Currently, one of the critical limitations of penile urethroplasty is the common need for a staged reconstruction with all the inconveniences for the patient, and a 20–31% incidence of graft failure following the first stage, which leads to further revision(s) prior to the final tubularization [95]. Insufficient oral mucosal grafts for panurethral stricture reconstruction, especially in redo cases, add serious problems.

Considerable research has been done in the areas of biomaterials, regenerative medicine, including scar modulation, and tissue engineering to overcome the limitations of current penile urethral stricture management. These experimental technologies appear exciting, revolutionary, and ripe with potential. The main goals of these research areas would be to produce scar inhibitors that might be placed into the stricture after urethrotomy, on the one hand, and to generate an ideal biomaterial in unlimited quantities, easily cultured in laboratory, readily available "off the shelf" and without the morbidity associated with graft harvesting, on the other hand. Unfortunately, we are not quite there yet.

10. Conclusion

The surgical treatment of penile urethral stricture is continually evolving. No one technique is appropriate for all situations, and the successful reconstructive urologist needs to be comfortable with a repertoire of different, versatile techniques in order to best treat each individual patient's problem. Since the early 1990s, OMG was introduced in urethral reconstructive surgery and has become the first choice of most urethral surgeons.

Although all are grouped as anterior urethral strictures, penile urethral strictures are different from bulbar urethral strictures. Flaps are still preferred to grafts in long, recurrent penile urethral strictures by some surgeons. Recently, one-stage dorsal OMG urethroplasty via perineal approach has been suggested for the management of most strictures of the penile shaft urethra with both good functional and remarkable cosmetic outcomes. However, in patients who have experienced failed hypospadias repair or in whom the penile skin and urethral plate are not suitable for urethroplasty, two-stage (usually multistage) urethroplasty is recommended. Management of some lengthy, complex strictures remains a great challenge even for experienced reconstructive surgeons. Staged urethroplasty, such as the Johanson's technique with or without the use of grafts, is still a good surgical option. Regenerative medicine continues to show promise, but further investigation is needed to reach clinical application in the future. All in all, these great improvements in penile urethral surgical technique should lead to optimization of the surgical treatment algorithm.

Author details

Francisco E. Martins[1*], Pedro Simoes de Oliveira[1] and Natalia M. Martins[2]

1 Department of Urology, School of Medicine, Santa Maria Hospital/CHULN, University of Lisbon, Lisbon, Portugal

2 Urology Unit, ULSNA, Portalegre, Portugal

*Address all correspondence to: faemartins@gmail.com

References

[1] Velasquez EF, Barreto JE, Cold CJ, Cubilla AL, et al. Penis and distal urethra. In: Mills SE, editor. Histology for Pathologists. Vol. 3. Philadelphia: Lippincott Williams and Wilkins; 2007. pp. 983-997

[2] Dagrosa LM, Gormley A. Anatomy of the urethra. In: Keane TE, Graham SD, editors. Glenn's Urologic Surgery. 8th ed. Philadelphia: Wolters Kluwer; 2016. pp. 311-314

[3] Fenton AS, Morey AF, Aviles R, et al. Anterior urethral strictures: Etiology and characteristics. Urology. 2005;**65**:1055-1058

[4] Lumen N, Hoebeke P, Willemsen P. Etiology of urethral stricture in the 21st century. The Journal of Urology. 2009;**182**:983-987

[5] Palminteri E, Berdondini E, Verze P, Nunzio CD, Vitarelli A, Carmignani L. Contemporary urethral stricture characteristic in the developed world. Urology. 2013;**81**:190-197

[6] Barbagli G, Lazzeri M, Palminteri E, Turini D. Lichen sclerosus of male genitalia involving anterior urethra. Lancet. 1999;**354**:429

[7] Pugliese JM, Morey AF, Peteron AC. Lichen sclerosus: Review of the literature and current recommendations for management. The Journal of Urology. 2007;**178**:2268-2276

[8] Elliott S, Brandes SB. Etiology, histology and classification of urethral stricture disease. In: Brandes SB, Morey AF, editors. Advanced Male Urethral and Genital Reconstructive Surgery. 2nd ed. NY: Humana Press; 2014. pp. 95-102

[9] Nuss GR, Granieri MA, Zhao LC. Presenting symptoms of anterior urethral stricture disease: A disease specific, patient reported questionnaire to measure outcomes. The Journal of Urology. 2012;**187**:559-562

[10] El-Ghar MA, Osman Y, Elbaz E, El-Diasty T. MR urethrogram versus combined retrograde urethrogram and sonourethrography in diagnosis of urethral stricture. European Journal of Radiology. 2010;**74**:193-198

[11] McAninch JW, Laing FC, Jeffrey RB Jr. Sonourethrography in the evaluation of the urethral strictures: A preliminary report. The Journal of Urology. 1988;**139**:294-297

[12] Nash PA, McAninch JW, Bruce JE. Sonourethrography in the evaluation of anterior urethral strictures. The Journal of Urology. 1995;**154**:72-76

[13] Sachse H. Treatment of urethral stricture: Transurethral slit in view using sharp section. Fortschritte der Medizin. 1974;**92**:12-15

[14] Steenkamp JW, Heyns CF, de Kock M. Internal urethrotomy versus dilatation ass treatment for male urethral strictures: A prospective, randomized comparison. The Journal of Urology. 1997;**157**:98-101

[15] Dubey D. The current role of direct vision internal urethrotomy and self-catheterization for anterior urethral strictures. Indian Journal of Urology. 2011;**27**:392-396

[16] Heyns CF, Steenkamp JW, de Kock ML, Whitaker P. Treatment of male urethral strictures: Is repeated dilatation or internal urethrotomy useful? The Journal of Urology. 1998;**160**:356-358

[17] Pansadoro V, Emiliozzi P. Internal urethrotomy in the management of anterior urethral strictures: Long-term

follow-up. The Journal of Urology. 1996;**156**:73-75

[18] Santucci R, Eisenberg L. Urethrotomy has a much lower success rate than previously reported. The Journal of Urology. 2010;**183**:1859-1862

[19] Naudé AM, Heyns CF. What is the place of internal urethrotomy in the treatment of urethral stricture disease? Nature Clinical Practice. Urology. 2005;**2**(11):538-545

[20] Gallegos MA, Santucci RA. Advances in urethral stricture management. F1000Research. 2016;**5**(F10000Faculty Rev):2913. DOI: 10.12688/f1000reearch.9741.1

[21] Jin T, Ki H, Jiang L-H Wang L, Wang K-J. Safety and efficacy of laser and cold knife urethrotomy for urethral stricture. Chinese Medical Journal. 2010;**123**:1589-1595

[22] Bürger RA et al. The buccal mucosa graft for urethral reconstruction: A preliminary report. The Journal of Urology. 1992;**147**:662-664

[23] Dessanti A, Rigamonti W, Merulla V, Falchetti D, Caccia G. Autologous buccal mucosa graft for hypospadia repair: An initial report. The Journal of Urology. 1992;**147**:1081-1084

[24] Lumen N, Oosterlinck W, Hoebeke P. Urethral reconstruction using buccal mucosa or penile skin grafts: Systematic review and meta-analysis. Urologia Internationalis. 2012;**89**:387-394

[25] Markiewicz MR et al. The oral mucosa graft: A systematic review. The Journal of Urology. 2007;**178**:387-394

[26] Barbagli G, Sansalone S, Djinovic R, Romano G, Lazzeri M. Current controversies in reconstructive surgery of the anterior urethra: A clinical overview. International Brazilian Journal of Urology. 2012;**38**:307-316

[27] Andrich DE, Leach CJ, Mundy AR. The Barbagli procedure gives the best results for patch urethroplasty of the bulbar urethra. BJU International. 2001;**88**:385-389

[28] Iselin CE, Webster GD. Dorsal onlay urethroplasty for urethral stricture repair. World Journal of Urology. 1998;**16**:181-185

[29] Wessells H. Ventral onlay graft techniques for urethroplasty. The Urologic Clinics of North America. 2002;**29**:381-387

[30] Elliot SP, Metro MJ, McAninch JW. Long-term follow-up of the ventrally placed buccal mucosa onlay graft in bulbar urethral reconstruction. The Journal of Urology. 2003;**169**:1754-1757

[31] Morey AF, McAninch JW. When and how to use buccal mucosal grafts in adult bulbar urethroplasty. Urology. 1996;**48**:194-198

[32] Blandy JP, Singh M, Notley RG, Treidder GC. The results and complications of scrotal-flap urethroplasty for stricture. British Journal of Urology. 1971;**43**:52-57

[33] Yachia D. A new, one-stage pedicled scrotal kin graft urethroplasty. The Journal of Urology. 1986;**136**(3):589-592

[34] Provet JA. Scrotal island flap urethroplasty in the management of bulbar urethral strictures. The Journal of Urology. 1989;**142**(6):1455-1457

[35] Gil-Vernet A, Arango O, Gil-Vernet J Jr, Gelabert-Mas A, Gil-Vernet J. Scrotal flap epilation in urethroplasty: Concepts and technique. The Journal of Urology. 1995;**154**(5):1723-1726

[36] Gil-Vernet J, Arango O, Gil-Vernet A, Gil-Vernet J Jr, Gelabert-Mas A. A new biaxial epilated scrotal flap for reconstructive urethral surgery. The Journal of Urology. 1997;**158**(2):412-420

[37] Orandi A. One-stage urethroplasty: 4-Year follow-up. The Journal of Urology. 1972;**107**(6):717-719

[38] Quartey KM. One-stage penile/preputial island flap urethroplasty for urethral stricture. The Journal of Urology. 1985;**134**(3):474-475

[39] McAninch JW. Reconstruction of extensive urethral strictures: Circular fasciocutaneous penile flap. The Journal of Urology. 1993;**149**(3):488-491

[40] Johanson B. Reconstruction of the male urethra in strictures. Application of the buried intact epithelium technique. Acta Chirurgica Scandinavica. 1953;**176**(Suppl. 176): 1-89

[41] Bracka A. Hypospadias repair: The two-stage alternative. British Journal of Urology. 1995;**76**(Suppl. 3):31-41

[42] Bracka A. A versatile two-stage hypospadias repair. British Journal of Plastic Surgery. 1995;**48**:345-352

[43] Bracka A. The role of two-stage repair in modern hypospadiology. Indian Journal of Urology. 2008;**24**:210-218

[44] Devine CJ, Franz JP, Horton CE. Evaluation and treatment of patients with failed hypospadias repair. The Journal of Urology. 1978;**119**:223-226

[45] Stecker JF, Horton CE, Devine CJ, McCraw JB. Hypospadias cripples. The Urologic Clinics of North America. 1981;**8**:539-544

[46] Barbagli G, De Angelis M, Palminteri E, Lazzeri M. Failed hypospadias repair presenting in adults. European Urology. 2006;**49**:887-895

[47] Tang S-H, Hammer CC, Doumanian L, Santucci RA. Adult urethral stricture disease after childhood hypospadias repair. Advances in Urology. 2008:150315. DOI: 10.1155/2008/150315

[48] Malone P. A new technique for meatal stenosis in patients with lichen sclerosus. The Journal of Urology. 2004;**172**:949-952

[49] Navalón P, Ramada C, Ordono F, Pallas Y, Monllor ME. Long-term follow-up of malone meatoplasty for meatal stenosis in patients with lichen sclerosus. Journal of Anesthesia and Surgery. 2016;**4**(2):121-124

[50] Cohney BC. A penile flap procedure for the relief of meatal strictures. British Journal of Urology. 1963;**35**:182-183

[51] Blandy JP, Tresider GC. Meatoplasty. British Journal of Urology. 1967;**39**:633-634

[52] Brannen GE. Meatal reconstruction. The Journal of Urology. 1976;**116**: 319-321

[53] De Sy WA. Aesthetic repair of meatal stricture. The Journal of Urology. 1984;**132**:678-679

[54] Jordan GH. Reconstruction of the fossa navicularis. The Journal of Urology. 1987;**138**:102-104

[55] Armenakas NA, Morey AF, McAninch JW. Reconstruction of the resistant strictures of the fossa navicularis and meatus. The Journal of Urology. 1998;**160**:359-363

[56] DeLong JM, Jordan GH. Reconstruction of the fossa navicularis. In: Smith JA Jr, Howards S, Preminger GM, Dmochowski RR, editors. Hinman's

Atlas of Urologic Surgery. 4th ed. Philadelphia: Elsevier; 2018. pp. 686-692

[57] Devine CJ, Horton CE. A one stage hypospadias repair. Journal of Urology. 2002;**167**:1169-1174 (reprinted from J Urol, 85: 166-172, 1961)

[58] Snodgrass W. Tubularized, incised plate urethroplasty for distal hypospadias. The Journal of Urology. 1994;**151**(2):464-465

[59] Asopa M, Garg M, Singhal GC, et al. Dorsal free graft urethroplasty for urethral stricture by ventral sagittal urethrotomy approach. Urology. 2001;**58**:657-659

[60] Gaur DD. Endourethral urethroplasty—Use of a new catheter. The Journal of Urology. 1983;**130**(5):905-908

[61] Naudé JH. Endoscopic skin-graft urethroplasty. World Journal of Urology. 1998;**16**(3):171-174

[62] Kuyumcuoglu U et al. Antegrade endourethroplasty with free skin graft for recurrent vesicourethral anastomotic strictures after radical prostatectomy. Journal of Endourology. 2010;**24**(1):63-67

[63] Seth A, Saini AK, Dogra PN. Hybrid minimally invasive urethroplasty for pan-anterior urethral strictures: Initial results. Urologia Internationalis. 2012;**89**(1):116-119

[64] Nikolavsky D, Abouelleil M, Daneshvar M. Transurethral ventral buccal mucosa graft inlay urethroplasty for reconstruction of fossa navicularis and distal urethral strictures: Surgical technique and preliminary results. International Urology and Nephrology. 2016;**48**:1823. DOI: 10.1007/s11255-016-1381-1

[65] Gelman J, Sohn W. One-stage repair of obliterative distal urethral strictures with buccal graft urethral plate reconstruction and simultaneous onlay penile skin flap. The Journal of Urology. 2011;**186**(3):935-938

[66] Tonkin JB, Jordan GH. Management of distal anterior urethral strictures. Nature Reviews. Urology. 2009;**6**:533-538

[67] Quartey JK. One-stage penile/preputial cutaneous island flap urethroplasty for urethral stricture: A preliminary report. The Journal of Urology. 1983;**129**(2):284-287

[68] Quartey JK. One-stage penile/preputial island flap urethroplasty for difficult posterior urethral strictures. World Journal of Urology. 1987;**5**:37-40

[69] Chapple C, Turner-Warwick. Substitution urethroplasty and the pedicle island skin procedure. In: McAninch JW, editor. Traumatic and Reconstructive Urology. Philadelphia: WB Saunders Company; 1996. pp. 571-594

[70] Devine PC, Horton CE, Devine CJ Sr, et al. Use of full thickness skin grafts in repair of urethral strictures. The Journal of Urology. 1963;**90**:67-71

[71] Barbagli G, Pellegrini G, Corradini F, Montorsi F, Sansalone S, Butnaru B, et al. One-stage penile urethroplasty using oral mucosa graft and glue. European Urology. 2006;**70**(6):1069-1075

[72] Martins FE, Oliveira T, Oliveira P, Felício J, Dave C, Martins NK. Perineal incision to repair penile urethral strictures is a versatile and cosmetic approach. In: Presented at the 37th Congress of the Societé Internationale d'Urologie; Lisbon, October 19-22. 2017

[73] Martins F, Kulkarni S, Joshi P, Marcelino J, de Oliveira TR, Oliveira P, et al. Kulkarni technique of perineal approach with penile inversion for

surgical repair of anterior urethral strictures: Functional and cosmetic outcomes. The Journal of Urology. 2016;**195**(Suppl. 4):e1001-e1002

[74] Kulkarni S, Barbagli G, Sansalone, Lazzeri M. One-sided anterior urethroplasty: A new dorsal onlay graft technique. BJU International. 2009;**104**(8):1150-1155

[75] Andrich DE, Greenwell TJ, Mundy AR. The problems of penile urethroplasty with particular reference to 2-tage reconstructions. The Journal of Urology. 2003;**170**:87-89

[76] Schreiter F, Noll F. Mesh graft urethroplasty using split thickness graft or foreskin. The Journal of Urology. 1989;**142**(5):1223-1226

[77] Carr LK, MacDiarmid SA, Webster GD. Treatment of complex anterior urethral stricture disease with mesh graft urethroplasty. The Journal of Urology. 1997;**157**(1):104-108

[78] Mori RL, Angermeier KW. Staged urethroplasty in the management of complex anterior urethral stricture disease. Translational Andrology and Urology. 2015;**4**(1):29-34

[79] Sinha RJ, Singh V, Sankhwar SN, Dalela D. Donor site morbidity in oral mucosa graft urethroplasty: Implications of tobacco consumption. BMC Urology. 2009;**9**:15

[80] Vacanti JP, Morse MA, Salzman WM, Domd AJ, Perez-Atayde A, Langer R. Selective cell transplantation using bioabsorbable artificial polymers as matrices. Journal of Pediatric Surgery. 1988;**23**:3-9

[81] Mangera A, Chapple CR. Tissue engineering in urethral reconstruction—An update. Asian Journal Andrology. 2013;**15**:89-92. DOI: 10.1038/aja.2012.91; published online 8 October 2012

[82] Bharadwaj S, Liu G, Shi Y, et al. Multipotent differentiation of human urine-derived stem cells: Potential for therapeutic applications in urology. Stem Cells. 2013;**13**(9):1840-1856

[83] Ikada Y. Challenges in tissue engineering. Journal of the Royal Society Interface. 2006;**3**:589-601

[84] Orabi H, AbouShwareb T, Zang Y, Yoo JJ, Atala A. Cell-seeded tubularized scaffolds for reconstruction of long urethral defects: A preclinical study. European Urology. 2013;**63**(3):531-538

[85] Karatas OF, Cimentepe E, Bayrak O, et al. A new application for urethral strictures: Tacrolimus-eluting stent. Journal of Endourology. 2010;**24**(6):1043-1044

[86] Shin JH, Song HY, Chai CG, et al. Tissue hyperplasia: Influence of a paclitaxel-eluting stent—Preliminary study in a canine urethral study. Radiology. 2005;**234**(2):438-444

[87] Spencer J, Blakely S, Daugherty M, Angulo JC, Martins F, Venkatesan K, et al. Clinical and patient-reported outcomes of 1-sided anterior urethroplasty for long-segment or panurethral strictures. Urology. 2018;**111**:208-213

[88] Coursey JW, Morey AF, McAninch JW, et al. Erectile function after anterior urethroplasty. Journal of Urology. 2001;**166**:2273-2276

[89] Erickson BA, Granieri MA, Meeks JJ, McVary KT, Gonzalez CM. Prospective analysis of ejaculatory function after anterior urethral reconstruction. The Journal of Urology. 2010;**184**:238-242

[90] Erickson BA, Granieri MA, Meeks JJ, Cashy JP, Gonzalez CM. Prospective analysis of erectile dysfunction after anterior urethroplasty: Incidence and

recovery of function. The Journal of Urology. 2010;**183**:657-661

[91] Patel DP, Elliott SP, Voelzke BB, Erickson BA, McClung CD, Presson AP, et al. Patient reported sexual function after staged penile urethroplasty. Urology. 2015;**86**(2):395-400

[92] Blaschko SD, Sanford MT, Cinman NM, McAninch JW, Breyer BN. De novo erectile dysfunction after anterior urethroplasty: A systematic review and meta-analysis. BJU International. 2013;**112**(5):655-663

[93] Granieri M, Webster G, Lentz A, Fraser A, Peterson A. Lower urinary tract symptoms associated with recurrence afterurethroplasstyfor anterior urethral stricture disease. The Journal of Urology. 2014;**191**(4S):e123

[94] Tao H, Jiang YY, Jun Q, Ding X, Jian DL, Jie D, et al. Analysis of risk factors leading to postoperative urethral stricture and bladder neck contracture following transurethral resection of prostate. International Brazilian Journal of Urology. 2016;**42**(2):302-311. DOI: 10.1590/S1677-5538.IBJU.2014.0500

[95] Campos-Juanatey F, Bugeja S, Ivaz SL, Frost A, Andrich DE, Mundy AR. Management of penile urethral strictures: Challenges and future directions. World Journal of Clinical Urology. 2016;**5**(1):1-10. ISSN: 2219-2816 (online)

[96] Jordan GH, McCammon KA. Surgery of the penis and urethra. In: Wein AJ, editor. Campbell-Walsh Urology. 10th ed. Philadelphia: Elsevier; 2012

[97] Armenakas NA, McAninch JW. Fossa navicularis and meatal stricture penile flap reconstruction. In: McAninch JW, editor. Traumatic and Reconstructive Urology. Philadelphia: W. B. Saunders Company; 1996

[98] Elliott SP, McAninch JW. Reconstruction of strictures of penile urethra. In: Smith JA Jr, Howards SS, Preminger GM, Dmochowski RR, editors. Hinman's Atlas of Urologic Surgery. 4th ed. Philadelphia: Elsevier; 2018

[99] McAninch JW. Fasciocutaneous penile flap in reconstruction of complex anterior urethral strictures. In: McAninch JW, editor. Traumatic and Reconstructive Urology. Philadelphia: W. B. Saunders Company; 1996

Chapter 7

Lower Urinary Tract Symptoms (LUTS) and Sexual Function and Dysfunction

Charalampos Konstantinidis, Ioannis Eleftheropoulos and Achileas Karafotias

Abstract

In recent years, the coexistence of sexual dysfunction (SD) and lower urinary tract symptoms (LUTS) has become a popular topic for researchers. Numerous clinical epidemiologic studies have been planned for this reason and have evaluated the relationship between these seemingly irrelevant urological conditions. The connection between SD and LUTS has already been acknowledged, and common pathophysiological pathways have been recognized. In this chapter was attempted to evaluate the impact on patient's quality of life (QoL), common pathophysiological pathways and therapy aspects of this condition. SD and LUTS are common problems among the general population and affect a great percentage of urological patients. It is a subject that affects the community in social, financial, and psychological terms. In this case, research for new treatment options has been triggered as phosphodiesterase type 5 inhibitors established their role as the widely approved combination therapy.

Keywords: lower urinary tract symptoms (LUTS), sexual dysfunction (SD), PDE5i

1. Introduction

In recent years, the coexistence of sexual dysfunction and lower urinary tract symptoms has become a popular topic for researchers. Numerous clinical epidemiologic studies have been planned for this reason and have evaluated the relationship between these seemingly irrelevant urological fields of study. In this chapter, an approach to these two fields, their impact on patients' quality of life (QoL), common pathophysiological pathways and therapy aspects are attempted. Both are common problems among the general population and affect a great percentage of urological patients. In this case, research for new treatment options has been triggered as phosphodiesterase type 5 inhibitors established their role as the widely approved combination therapy.

2. Lower urinary tract symptoms

Lower urinary tract symptoms (LUTS) are a common complaint in adult men and women with a major impact on quality of life (QoL) [1–4]. They can be divided into storage, voiding, and postmicturition symptoms [5]. LUTS are strongly associated with aging [1, 2] and also with a number of modifiable risk factors, suggesting potential targets for prevention (e.g., metabolic syndrome) [6]. Most elderly men have at least one LUTS [2], which is often mild or not very bothersome [4, 7, 8]. LUTS progression is a dynamic procedure. LUTS may persist and upscale over long time periods, or they may retreat [2]. LUTS have usually been related to bladder outlet obstruction (BOO), which is often caused by an increase of prostatic volume, as a result of benign prostate hyperplasia (BPH) [3, 5]. On the contrary, numerous studies have shown that LUTS are often not related to the BPH [2, 9]. Bladder dysfunction may also cause LUTS, such as detrusor overactivity or overactive bladder syndrome (OAB), detrusor underactivity, and structural or functional abnormalities of the urinary tract and its surrounding tissues [9]. Prostatitis may also cause the appearance of LUTS [10, 11]. Furthermore, there are some nonurological conditions that may be related to urinary symptoms, mainly to nocturia [2].

The definitions of the most common conditions related to LUTS are presented below:

- Acute retention of urine is defined as a painful and palpable bladder when the patient cannot urinate [5].

- Chronic retention of urine is defined as a nonpainful bladder, which remains palpable even though the patient has urinated. It may also be accompanied by incontinence [5].

- Bladder outlet obstruction (BOO) is characterized by reduced urine flow rate and increased detrusor pressure. It can be diagnosed by studying the synchronous values of detrusor pressure and urine flow rate [5].

- Benign prostatic obstruction (BPO) is a form of BOO, diagnosed when the cause of outlet obstruction is known to be BPH [5].

- Detrusor overactivity (DO) is a urodynamic observation characterized by involuntary detrusor contractions during the bladder filling phase [5].

- Overactive bladder (OAB) syndrome is characterized by urinary urgency, with or without urinary incontinence, usually with increased daytime frequency and nocturia, and in this case, there is no proven infection or other obvious pathology [12].

Patient's history must be assessed thoroughly [13–15]. A medical history aims to identify relevant comorbidities and potential causes, including medical and neurological diseases. Lifestyle habits, medication, emotional, and psychological factors must also be reviewed. When relevant, the sexual function should be assessed, preferably with validated symptom questionnaires such as the International Index for Erectile Function (IIEF). The literature recommends, for male LUTS assessment, the use of validated symptom score questionnaire [13, 15]. Several questionnaires have been developed, which are sensitive to symptom changes. In this case, they are helpful in monitoring treatment approaches [16–22]. Symptom scores are helpful in quantifying LUTS and identifying the predominant symptoms. Nevertheless, they are not disease- or age specific.

3. Sexual dysfunction

It is difficult to identify the prevalence of sexual dysfunction in men, because there is no standard definition of sexual dysfunction (SD). Erectile dysfunction

(ED) is defined as the persistent inability to attain and maintain an erection sufficient to permit satisfactory sexual performance [23]. Penile erection is a complex phenomenon, which implies coordination among the neurological, vascular, and smooth muscle compartment. It includes arterial dilation, trabecular smooth muscle relaxation, and activation of the corporal veno-occlusive mechanism [24]. ED may affect physical and psychosocial health. It might have a significant impact on the QoL of sufferers and their partners' as well [25–27]. Therefore, ED should not be regarded only as a QoL issue, but also as a potential warning sign of cardiovascular disease (CVD), as it can be an early manifestation of coronary artery and peripheral vascular disease [28–30].

The pathophysiology of ED may be vasculogenic, neurogenic, anatomical, hormonal, drug-induced, and/or psychogenic [24]. Usually, many pathophysiology pathways can be comorbid and concomitant, negatively impacting on erectile function. In most cases, ED is the result of more than one organic pathophysiological element and, very often, a psychological component. ED was initially classified into three categories based on its etiology. These include organic, psychogenic, and mixed ED. Nowadays, these are recognized as two categories: the psychogenic and the mixed one, as any organic ED has an additional psychogenic impact that interferes with the pathophysiology of ED and causes additional distress to the patient.

Epidemiological data have shown a high incidence and prevalence of ED worldwide. The Massachusetts male aging study (MMAS) [25] reported, in noninstitutionalized men aged 40–70 years in the Boston area, an overall prevalence of 52% ED. Prevalence for minimal, moderate, and complete ED was 17.2, 25.2, and 9.6%, respectively. In the Cologne study of men aged 30–80 years, the prevalence of ED was 19.2% [65]. The incidence rate of ED (new cases per 1000 men annually) was 26 in the long-term data from the MMAS study [66] and 19.2 (mean follow-up of 4.2 years) in a Dutch study [31].

ED shares common risk factors with CVD (e.g., obesity, diabetes mellitus, dyslipidemia, metabolic syndrome, lack of exercise, and smoking) [27, 32–34]. The association among ED and age, diabetes mellitus, body mass index (BMI) [35, 36], obstructive sleep apnea, and hyperhomocysteinemia has been established [37–39]. A number of studies have shown evidence that lifestyle modification [29, 40] and pharmacotherapy [40, 41] for CVD risk factors may also improve sexual function in men with ED. Epidemiological studies have also demonstrated consistent evidence for an association between LUTS and sexual dysfunction, regardless of age, other comorbidities, and behavioral factors [42]. The multinational survey on the aging male (MSAM-7) study (performed in France, Germany, Spain, Italy, the Netherlands, the USA, and the UK) investigated the relationship between LUTS and sexual dysfunction in over 12,000 men aged 50–80 years. From 83% of sexually active men, the prevalence of LUTS was 90%, with the prevalence of ED being 49%. The complete absence of erection was reported in 10% of patients. The prevalence of ejaculatory disorders has been reported in 46% of patients [43]. Association between chronic prostatitis or chronic pelvic pain syndrome (CP/CPPS) and ED is confirmed [44].

Surgical interventions to the prostate also have an impact on erectile function according to the type of surgery that was performed [45]. Epidemiologically, there are other risk factors that potentially associate to ED, including psoriasis [46–48], gouty arthritis [49, 50], ankylosing spondylitis [51], nonalcoholic fatty liver [52], chronic liver disorders [53], chronic periodontitis [54], open-angle glaucoma [55], inflammatory bowel disease [56], and complications following transrectal ultrasound (TRUS) guided prostate biopsy [57].

World Health Organization (WHO) and International Classifications of Diseases-10 (ICD-10) define female sexual dysfunction as "the various ways in which an individual is unable to participate in a sexual relationship as she would wish" [58]. There are three categories of sexual dysfunction: female sexual interest-arousal disorder, female orgasmic disorder, and genito-pelvic pain-penetration disorder [59]. It is estimated that 10% of women suffer from female sexual interest-arousal disorder and 3.5–35% present orgasmic problems [60].

Validated psychometric questionnaires, such as the International Index for Erectile Function (IIEF) [61] or the sexual health inventory for men (SHIM) [62], are the assessment tools needed in different sexual function domains (i.e., erectile function, sexual desire, intercourse, orgasmic function, and overall satisfaction), as well as for the potential impact of a specific treatment modality. The use of the erectile hardness score for the assessment of penile rigidity in practice and in clinical trial research is supported by psychometric analyses [63]. Patients should be screened for symptoms of possible hypogonadism (testosterone deficiency), libido, fatigue, cognitive impairment, and LUTS. Even though LUTS does not represent a contraindication to treat a patient for late-onset hypogonadism, screening for LUTS severity is clinically relevant [64].

4. The relationship between ED and LUTS

A lot of epidemiological studies demonstrate the coexistence of ED and LUTS. It is also proven that the existence of LUTS is a risk factor for ED. The patient's age and the severity of LUTS are independent prognostic factors for ED, as well. Although it is not clear if LUTS lead to ED, or ED results to LUTS, or these conditions are just coexisting, their relation is very narrow and clear, especially in older patients. Therefore, men who suffer from LUTS should be checked for ED and men who present ED should be evaluated for LUTS. There are four theories that try to correlate LUTS with ED. These theories include deregulation of NO/NOS system, increased sympathetic tone (autonomic hyperactivity (AH)), up-regulation of Rho-kinase, and chronic hypoxia. Common vascular risk factors can combine and support these theories.

4.1 Alteration in nitric oxide (NO)

The role of nitric oxide (NO) in erectile function is well known as the main regulator of penile corporal smooth muscle relaxation and resultant erection. The decrease in NO/cyclic guanosine monophosphate (cGMP) has the effect of reduction in NO synthase (NOS) due to endothelial dysfunction. Luck or reduction of smooth muscle relaxation of the bladder neck, prostate and urethra may lead to LUTS. The NO system has been shown to be down-regulated in the transition zone of the prostate in BPH when compared with normal controls [67, 68].

4.2 Autonomic hyperactivity (AH)

AH, as a component of the metabolic syndrome, refers to dysregulation of sympathetic and parasympathetic tone. Increased sympathetic tone results in flaccidity and antagonizes penile erection, due to vasoconstriction. Parasympathetic activation can lead to prostate smooth muscle contraction (due to activation of the M2 receptors), so nonrelaxing bladder neck, prostatic urethra, and pelvic floor may lead to LUTS [67, 68].

4.3 RhoA/rho-kinase-calcium-sensitizing pathway

Smooth muscle tone is adjusted commonly not only through the calcium-dependent mechanism, but also through the activity of RhoA/ROCK calcium pathway. Activation of RhoA-ROCK pathway can affect smooth muscle relaxation and finally increase ED and LUTS. Therefore, penile RhoA/ROCK signaling was increased in pathologic situations associated with ED, like diabetes and involuntary bladder contractions were associated with increased signaling of the muscarinic receptor-activated RhoA/ROCK pathway. Increase in RhoA/ROCK was demonstrated in corpora cavernosa and bladder of spontaneously hypertensive rats (SHR), a rat strain genetically prone to develop BPH and OAB. The inhibition of ROCK reduces bladder hyperactivity, limits contractions in bladder strips from SHR, and improves erectile function [67, 68].

4.4 Pelvic atherosclerosis

Atherosclerosis of the bladder, prostate, and penis serves an extra assumption linking LUTS with ED. The theory claims that the risks for ED (smoking, hypertension, hypercholesterolemia, and diabetes mellitus) also affect on LUTS. An epidemiologic study was published that supports this theory, all men and women who had two risk factors of atherosclerosis (diabetes mellitus, hypertension, hyperlipidemia, and nicotine use) and had a statistically higher International Prostate Symptom Score (IPSS) compared with those with one or no risk factors at all. Smooth muscle changes in the prostate, bladder, and penis of animal models of hypercholesterolemia and pelvic ischemia are quite similar. Hypoxia drives to overexpression of TGFb1, and converted prostanoid production has been suggested as potential mechanisms. Similarly, penile ischemia leads to smooth muscle loss in it and ends up with ED. Likewise, the loss of smooth muscle in the bladder may decrease compliance and increase the symptoms of LUTS. Additionally, bladder ischemia either from BOO or pelvic vascular disease would result in bladder smooth muscle loss with the resultant replacement of collagen deposition and fibrosis as well as loss of compliance, overactivity, and impaired contractility. Loss of smooth muscle in the prostate can induce a less distensible urethra, a decreased urinary flow rate, increased flow resistance, and worsening LUTS. Pelvic atherosclerosis associated with the previously described theories, as pelvic ischemia/atherosclerosis is a component of the metabolic syndrome/AH, up-regulates Rk activity, and reduces NOS expression. [35, 67, 68].

5. Multifactorial interaction between LUTS and ED

LUTS are significant indicators of a disease when the patient, caregiver, or partner realizes it, and change of them may lead him/her to find help from professionals. It is also known (from the 6th International Consultation on Incontinence 2016) that from overall world's population, 46% (of the adults >20 years) experience LUTS, 11.8% suffer from OAB symptoms, 8% complain of some type of urinary incontinence (UI), and 4% of severe stress urinary incontinence (SUI). Urinary incontinence is associated with reduced QoL, higher rates of depression, reduced work productivity, and decreased enjoyment of sexual activity [35, 69].

It is well known that sexual life, behavior, and relationships are very important for a good and healthy life, and they are affected by attitudes, social models and overall health. For sexual health many aspects are necessary and not only the absence of infirmity, disease or dysfunction. Sexual practice and habits have changed a lot over the last years, it is over also known that the sexual frequency and different practices are reducing with age. On the other hand, some sexual behaviors are more common in our days, like anal sex. These changes are more likely to be attributed to educational status, rather than economic status [69].

From a physiological prospect, the functions of pelvic organ functions are related as there is a direct relationship with the neuronal network of the pelvis that includes bladder, bowel, and sexual functions. Furthermore, vascular, hormonal, cellular, and other factors comprehensively affect pelvic organ functions. LUTS and ED in males share common pathophysiological pathways [4].

6. Effects of LUTS/incontinence on male sexual function: epidemiological data

Many large studies over the last years have proved the coexistence of SD in men with storage and voiding LUTS. Statistics from the Health Improvement Network database showed that from 11,327 men in the UK, there was a rise in the overall prevalence of recorded SD from 1.7% in 2000 to 4.9% in 2007. The odds ratio (OR) for ED was 3.0 (2.6–3.4) for storage LUTS, 2.6 (2.4–2.7) for voiding LUTS, and 4.0 (3.4–4.8) for voiding and storage LUTS. The EpiLUTS study (a cross-sectional, population-representative survey in the UK, Sweden, and the USA with 6326 men) show off an impact of OAB on sexual health. Both OAB wet and OAB dry were associated with poor sexual health, diminished enjoyment of sex ($P < 0.0001$), and decreased sexual activity. OAB dry/wet was very significant predictors of ED and ejaculatory dysfunction (EjD) in men. According to a study by Rosen et al., the attendance and severity of LUTS are independent risk factors for SD in older men [69].

LUTS are common in older men. While LUTS have a multifactorial etiology, BOO/BPH has traditionally been considered as one of the most common causes of LUTS. These symptoms, which include dribbling and urgency with leaking, nocturia, and difficulty in urinating, can also impact the sexual function, probably due to impact on QoL [70].

7. Medical and surgical therapy for LUTS and its impact on sexual function

The efficacy of all currently available treatments for LUTS is well studied. However, the negative impact of them on erectile function is under evaluation. Behavior modification therapies and phytotherapies seem to have minimal or no impact on sexual function, and even less efficacy on LUTS treatment. On the other hand, α-blockers, 5α-reductase inhibitors, and prostatic surgery are associated with improvement in LUTS, but they usually have a negative impact on the sexual function [68]. Many clinical trials have reported on the efficacy of chronic treatment with phosphodiesterase type 5 inhibitors (PDE5-Is), either alone or in combination with other therapies, in treating LUTS in men with or without ED [71].

α-Blockers such as alfuzosin, doxazosin, tamsulosin, and silodosin have shown similar efficacy, but their effect on sexual function is variable. They seem to have a slightly positive impact on erectile function. However, they can have a negative impact on orgasmic function and ejaculation [72]. Originally, the abnormal ejaculate was thought to be retrograde. However, it seems likely to be due to a decrease or absence of seminal fluid, possibly by a central effect. α-Blockers decrease the prostate secretion and inhibit the contraction of seminal vesicles as both effects are mediated by the sympathetic adrenergic system.

5α-Reductase inhibitors (5-ARIs) are usually offered to men with LUTS who have a prostate estimated to be larger than 40 ml and who are considered to be at high risk of progression [73–75]. Compared to α-blockers, 5-ARIs have a greater impact on sexual function. The side effects most frequently notified are reduced libido, ED, and ejaculation disorders such as dry orgasm, ejaculation failure, or decreased semen volume [76–78]. It must be mentioned that the effect of 5-ARIs on ejaculatory function is currently poorly studied.

Regarding surgical options, transurethral resection of the prostate (TURP) and transurethral incision of the prostate (TUIP) are the gold standard surgical techniques for BPH/BOO treatment. Dry orgasm after these operations ranges from 30.4 to 96.9% and 6.1 to 55.1%, respectively. Heterogeneous data are reported, mainly because only a few studies analyzed these rates [79–81] in a prospective fashion. ED has been found ranging from 3.4 to 32.4% [80, 81] after TURP.

Laser procedures, such as GreenLight photoselective vaporization of the prostate (PVP) and holmium laser enucleation of the prostate (HoLEP) are widely offered for BOO/BPH as well. The impact of GreenLight on sexual function seems to be close to that of TURP. One single study, comparing these two prostatic surgery techniques, reported no significant difference in the rate of retrograde ejaculation [82]. There is also no difference reported between TURP and PVP for erectile function [83, 84]. HoLEP seems to have comparable results. Specifically, the incidence of retrograde ejaculation and erectile dysfunction is comparable between HoLEP and TURP [85, 86]. It is reported that almost 75% of sexually active patients have retrograde ejaculation after HoLEP. Currently, both GreenLight and HoLEP surgeons are trying to develop ejaculation preserving techniques [87, 88].

Transurethral thermotherapy and microwave techniques such as transurethral needle ablation (TUNA) seem to have lower rates of retrograde ejaculation comparing to TURP. A few studies report that the incidence of retrograde ejaculation seems to be much lower compared to TURP, with no reported cases in the TUNA cohort, compared to the 45% of the TURP arm [89–91]. Urolift/prostatic urethral lift (PUL) is an alternative option and has shown positive results in terms of sexual function [92].

Currently, because of the increase in life expectancy, patients with LUTS often wish to preserve or to improve their sexual function according to their treatments. Physicians may focus on the symptoms without considering patients' wishes and expectations. In those cases, despite successful treatment, many patients still complain about their QoL due to the procedure or medication side effects.

8. Medical therapy for ED and its impact on LUTS

Phosphodiesterase type 5 (PDE5) is expressed in the whole of the lower urinary tract, including the urethra, prostate, and bladder. All these organs are targets of PDE5-Is [93–96]. PDE5 is prominently localized in the stroma and in the vascular bed (endothelial and smooth muscle cells), suggesting the action of PDE5-I on smooth muscle contraction and blood flow.

McVary et al. [97], in 2007, evaluated the safety and efficacy of tadalafil for the treatment of LUTS in men with or without ED, for the first time. A total of 479 patients were screened. After a 4-week washout and 4-week placebo run-in period, 281 were randomly assigned to a 6-week treatment with once-daily placebo or tadalafil 5 mg. After 6 weeks, the remaining 261 patients were assigned to continue with placebo for another 6 weeks (a total of 12 weeks of once-daily placebo treatment) or to dose escalate tadalafil to 20 mg once daily. Of 143 placebo-assigned patients, 121 (84.6%) were sexually active, 84 (59.2%) had no erectile dysfunction, and 76 (53.1%) were sexually active despite ED. On the other hand, 138 men treated with 5 or 20 mg tadalafil, 107 (77.5%) were sexually active, 99 (71.7%) had normal sexual function, and 80 (58.0%) were sexually active despite ED. The IPSS (including the IPSS-QoL question) and BII questionnaires were used in order to evaluate LUTS. Maximum urinary flow rate (Q_{max}) and average urinary flow rate (Q_{ave}) of free uroflowmetry were record and post-void residual urine (PVR) was measured by ultrasound after uroflowmetry. The erectile function (EF) domain of the International Index of Erectile Function (IIEF) questionnaire (questions 1–5 and 15) was used to estimate the sexual function.

Since 2007, numerous studies proved the safety and efficacy of PDE5s as a medical therapy for both LUTS and ED. Bora Irer et al. [98] studied LUTS, nocturia, SD, and the status of QoL in men with obstructive sleep apnea syndrome (OSAS). Patients applied continuous positive airway pressure (CPAP) treatment, which is one of the most effective treatments for OSAS, supplying positive air pressure for the opening of the respiratory tract and keeping high saturation of oxygen. Changes in IPSS, IIEF, Overactive Bladder Syndrome Score (OABSS), International Consultation on Incontinence Questionnaire for Male LUTS (ICIQ-MLUTS), Neuro-quality of life score (Nqol), 36-item Short Form Health Survey (SF-36), and Benign Prostatic Hyperplasia Impact Index (BII); the frequency of nocturia; and night-time urine volume were reported. After CPAP treatment, significant changes and improvements on these symptoms and QoL were observed. It has been shown that the frequency of nocturia decreases and erectile function and QoL improves in patients with OSAS under CPAP treatment [99, 100].

9. Conclusion

SD and LUTS are confirmed to have a strong connection. It is implied by common pathophysiological paths that seem to link these two complications, which have a great impact on a significant percentage of urological patients. For men, PDE5s inhibitors are the milestone of medical treatment for ED and LUTS. Their safety and efficacy are widely accepted. More studies need to support this relatively new field of research for both LUTS and SD, and new treatments may be used as an alternative in near future.

Author details

Charalampos Konstantinidis[1,2]*, Ioannis Eleftheropoulos[2] and Achileas Karafotias[2]

1 Urology and Neuro-Urology Unit, National Rehabilitation Center, Athens, Greece

2 Urology Department, General Hospital "Asklepieio Voulas", Athens, Greece

*Address all correspondence to: konstantinidischaralampos@yahoo.com

References

[1] Kupelian V et al. Prevalence of lower urinary tract symptoms and effect on quality of life in a racially and ethnically diverse random sample: The Boston area community health (BACH) survey. Archives of Internal Medicine. 2006;**166**:2381 https://www.ncbi.nlm.nih.gov/pubmed/17130393

[2] Agarwal A et al. What is the most bothersome lower urinary tract symptom? Individual- and population-level perspectives for both men and women. European Urology. 2014;**65**:1211 https://www.ncbi.nlm.nih.gov/pubmed/24486308

[3] De Ridder D et al. Urgency and other lower urinary tract symptoms in men aged >/= 40 years: A Belgian epidemiological survey using the ICIQ-MLUTS questionnaire. International Journal of Clinical Practice. 2015;**69**:358 https://www.ncbi.nlm.nih.gov/pubmed/25648652

[4] Taub DA et al. The economics of benign prostatic hyperplasia and lower urinary tract symptoms in the United States. Current Urology Reports. 2006;7:272 https://www.ncbi.nlm.nih.gov/pubmed/16930498

[5] Chapple C, Abrams P. Lower Urinary Tract Symptoms (LUTS): An International Consultation On Male LUTS. Societe Internationale d'Urologie (SIU). ISBN: 978-0-9877465-4-2

[6] Chapple CR et al. Lower urinary tract symptoms revisited: A broader clinical perspective. European Urology. 2008;**54**:563 https://www.ncbi.nlm.nih.gov/pubmed/18423969

[7] Gacci M et al. Metabolic syndrome and benign prostatic enlargement: A systematic review and meta-analysis. BJU International. 2015;**115**:24 https://www.ncbi.nlm.nih.gov/pubmed/24602293

[8] Ficarra V et al. The role of inflammation in lower urinary tract symptoms (LUTS) due to benign prostatic hyperplasia (BPH) and its potential impact on medical therapy. Current Urology Reports. 2014;**15**:463 https://www.ncbi.nlm.nih.gov/pubmed/25312251

[9] He Q et al. Metabolic syndrome, inflammation and lower urinary tract symptoms: Possible translational links. Prostate Cancer and Prostatic Diseases. 2016;**19**:7 https://www.ncbi.nlm.nih.gov/pubmed/26391088

[10] Drake MJ. Do we need a new definition of the overactive bladder syndrome? ICI-RS 2013. Neurourology and Urodynamics. 2014;**33**:622 http://www.ncbi.nlm.nih.gov/pubmed/24838519

[11] Novara G et al. Critical review of guidelines for BPH diagnosis and treatment strategy. European Urology Supplements. 2006;**4**:418 http://eu-acme.org/europeanurology/upload_articles/Novara2.pdf

[12] McVary KT et al. Update on AUA guideline on the management of benign prostatic hyperplasia. The Journal of Urology. 2011;**185**:1793 https://www.ncbi.nlm.nih.gov/pubmed/21420124

[13] Bosch J et al. Etiology, patient assessment and predicting outcome from therapy. International Consultation on Urological Diseases Male LUTS Guideline. 2013;**2013**:37

[14] Martin RM et al. Lower urinary tract symptoms and risk of prostate cancer: The HUNT 2 cohort, Norway. International Journal of Cancer. 2008;**123**:1924 https://www.ncbi.nlm.nih.gov/pubmed/18661522

[15] Young JM et al. Are men with lower urinary tract symptoms at increased risk

of prostate cancer? A systematic review and critique of the available evidence. BJU International. 2000;**85**:1037 https://www.ncbi.nlm.nih.gov/pubmed/10848691

[16] Donovan JL et al. Scoring the short form ICS male SF questionnaire. International continence society. The Journal of Urology. 2000;**164**:1948 https://www.ncbi.nlm.nih.gov/pubmed/11061889

[17] Epstein RS et al. Validation of a new quality of life questionnaire for benign prostatic hyperplasia. Journal of Clinical Epidemiology. 1992;**45**:1431 https://www.ncbi.nlm.nih.gov/pubmed/1281223

[18] Homma Y et al. Symptom assessment tool for overactive bladder syndrome--overactive bladder symptom score. Urology. 2006;**68**:318 https://www.ncbi.nlm.nih.gov/pubmed/16904444

[19] Schou J et al. The value of a new symptom score (DAN-PSS) in diagnosing uro-dynamic infravesical obstruction in BPH. Scandinavian Journal of Urology and Nephrology. 1993;**27**:489 https://www.ncbi.nlm.nih.gov/pubmed/7512747

[20] Homma Y et al. Core lower urinary tract symptom score (CLSS) questionnaire: A reliable tool in the overall assessment of lower urinary tract symptoms. International Journal of Urology. 2008;**15**:816 https://www.ncbi.nlm.nih.gov/pubmed/18657204

[21] D'Silva KA et al. Does this man with lower urinary tract symptoms have bladder outlet obstruction?: The rational clinical examination: A systematic review. JAMA. 2014;**312**:535 https://www.ncbi.nlm.nih.gov/pubmed/25096693

[22] Bryan NP et al. Frequency volume charts in the assessment and evaluation of treatment: How should we use them? European Urology. 2004;**46**:636 https://www.ncbi.nlm.nih.gov/pubmed/15474275

[23] Salonia A et al. Is erectile dysfunction a reliable proxy of general male health status? The case for the international index of erectile function-erectile function domain. The Journal of Sexual Medicine. 2012;**9**:2708 https://www.ncbi.nlm.nih.gov/pubmed/22897643

[24] Fisher WA et al. Erectile dysfunction (ED) is a shared sexual concern of couples I: Couple conceptions of ED. The Journal of Sexual Medicine. 2009;**6**:2746 https://www.ncbi.nlm.nih.gov/pubmed/19694926

[25] Dong JY et al. Erectile dysfunction and risk of cardiovascular disease: Meta-analysis of prospective cohort studies. Journal of the American College of Cardiology. 2011;**58**:1378 https://www.ncbi.nlm.nih.gov/pubmed/21920268

[26] Gandaglia G et al. A systematic review of the association between erectile dysfunction and cardiovascular disease. European Urology. 2014;**65**:968 https://www.ncbi.nlm.nih.gov/pubmed/24011423

[27] Gupta BP et al. The effect of lifestyle modification and cardiovascular risk factor reduction on erectile dysfunction: A systematic review and meta-analysis. Archives of Internal Medicine. 2011;**171**:1797 https://www.ncbi.nlm.nih.gov/pubmed/21911624

[28] Braun M et al. Epidemiology of erectile dysfunction: Results of the 'Cologne male survey. International Journal of Impotence Research. 2000;**12**:305 https://www.ncbi.nlm.nih.gov/pubmed/11416833

[29] Johannes CB et al. Incidence of erectile dysfunction in men 40 to 69

years old: Longitudinal results from the Massachusetts male aging study. The Journal of Urology. 2000;**163**:460 https://www.ncbi.nlm.nih.gov/pubmed/10647654

[30] Schouten BW et al. Incidence rates of erectile dysfunction in the Dutch general population. Effects of definition, clinical relevance and duration of follow-up in the Krimpen study. International Journal of Impotence Research. 2005;**17**:58 https://www.ncbi.nlm.nih.gov/pubmed/15510192

[31] Jackson G et al. Cardiovascular aspects of sexual medicine. The Journal of Sexual Medicine. 2010;**7**:1608 https://www.ncbi.nlm.nih.gov/pubmed/20388161

[32] Binmoammar TA et al. The impact of poor glycaemic control on the prevalence of erectile dysfunction in men with type 2 diabetes mellitus: A systematic review. Journal of the Royal Society of Medicine Open. 2016;**7**:2054270415622602 https://www.ncbi.nlm.nih.gov/pubmed/26981254

[33] Glina S et al. Modifying risk factors to prevent and treat erectile dysfunction. The Journal of Sexual Medicine. 2013;**10**:115 https://www.ncbi.nlm.nih.gov/pubmed/22971247

[34] Vlachopoulos C et al. Erectile dysfunction in the cardiovascular patient. European Heart Journal. 2013;**34**:2034 https://www.ncbi.nlm.nih.gov/pubmed/23616415

[35] Seftel AD et al. Coexisting lower urinary tract symptoms and erectile dysfunction: A systematic review of epidemiological data. International Journal of Clinical Practice. 2013;**67**:32 https://www.ncbi.nlm.nih.gov/pubmed/23082930

[36] Rosen R et al. Lower urinary tract symptoms and male sexual dysfunction: The multinational survey of the aging male (MSAM-7). European Urology. 2003;**44**:637 https://www.ncbi.nlm.nih.gov/pubmed/14644114

[37] Molina Leyva A et al. Sexual dysfunction in psoriasis: A systematic review. Journal of the European Academy of Dermatology and Venereology. 2015;**29**:649 https://www.ncbi.nlm.nih.gov/pubmed/25424331

[38] Fan D et al. Male sexual dysfunction and ankylosing spondylitis: A systematic review and metaanalysis. The Journal of Rheumatology. 2015;**42**:252 https://www.ncbi.nlm.nih.gov/pubmed/25448789

[39] Duman DG et al. Nonalcoholic fatty liver disease is associated with erectile dysfunction: A prospective pilot study. The Journal of Sexual Medicine. 2016;**13**:383 https://www.ncbi.nlm.nih.gov/pubmed/26853046

[40] Salonia A et al. Prevention and management of postprostatectomy sexual dysfunctions part 2: Recovery and preservation of erectile function, sexual desire, and orgasmic function. European Urology. 2012;**62**:273 https://www.ncbi.nlm.nih.gov/pubmed/22575910

[41] Salonia A et al. Prevention and management of postprostatectomy sexual dysfunctions. Part 1: Choosing the right patient at the right time for the right surgery. European Urology. 2012;**62**:261 https://www.ncbi.nlm.nih.gov/pubmed/22575909

[42] Sanda MG et al. Quality of life and satisfaction with outcome among prostate-cancer survivors. The New England Journal of Medicine. 2008;**358**:1250 https://www.ncbi.nlm.nih.gov/pubmed/18354103

[43] Schauer I et al. Have rates of erectile dysfunction improved within the past

17 years after radical prostatectomy? A systematic analysis of the control arms of prospective randomized trials on penile rehabilitation. Andrology. 2015;**3**:661 https://www.ncbi.nlm.nih.gov/pubmed/26198796

[44] Ficarra V et al. Systematic review and meta-analysis of studies reporting potency rates after robot- assisted radical prostatectomy. European Urology. 2012;**62**:418 https://www.ncbi.nlm.nih.gov/pubmed/22749850

[45] Stolzenburg JU et al. Effect of surgical approach on erectile function recovery following bilateral nerve-sparing radical prostatectomy: An evaluation utilising data from a randomised, double-blind, double-dummy multicentre trial of tadalafil vs placebo. BJU International. 2015;**116**:241 https://www.ncbi.nlm.nih.gov/pubmed/25560809

[46] Haglind E et al. Urinary incontinence and erectile dysfunction after robotic versus open radical prostatectomy: A prospective, controlled, nonrandomised trial. European Urology. 2015;**68**:216 https://www.ncbi.nlm.nih.gov/pubmed/25770484

[47] Yaxley JW et al. Robot-assisted laparoscopic prostatectomy versus open radical retropubic prostatectomy: Early outcomes from a randomised controlled phase 3 study. Lancet. 2016;**388**:1057 https://www.ncbi.nlm.nih.gov/pubmed/27474375

[48] Isgoren A et al. Erectile function outcomes after robot-assisted radical prostatectomy: Is it superior to open retropubic or laparoscopic approach. Sexual Medicine Reviews. 2014;**2**: 10-23. https://www.ncbi.nlm.nih.gov/pubmed/27784540

[49] Glickman L et al. Changes in continence and erectile function between 2 and 4 years after radical prostatectomy. The Journal of Urology. 2009;**181**:731 https://www.ncbi.nlm.nih.gov/pubmed/19091349

[50] Incrocci L et al. Pelvic radiotherapy and sexual function in men and women. The Journal of Sexual Medicine. 2013;**10**(Suppl 1):53 https://www.ncbi.nlm.nih.gov/pubmed/23387912

[51] Stember DS et al. The concept of erectile function preservation (penile rehabilitation) in the patient after brachytherapy for prostate cancer. Brachytherapy. 2012;**11**:87 https://www.ncbi.nlm.nih.gov/pubmed/22330103

[52] Cordeiro ER et al. High-intensity focused ultrasound (HIFU) for definitive treatment of prostate cancer. BJU International. 2012;**110**:1228 https://www.ncbi.nlm.nih.gov/pubmed/22672199

[53] Williams SB et al. Comparative effectiveness of cryotherapy vs brachytherapy for localised prostate cancer. BJU International. 2012;**110**:E92 https://www.ncbi.nlm.nih.gov/pubmed/22192688

[54] Hatzichristou D et al. Diagnosing sexual dysfunction in men and women: Sexual history taking and the role of symptom scales and questionnaires. The Journal of Sexual Medicine. 2016;**13**:1166 https://www.ncbi.nlm.nih.gov/pubmed/27436074

[55] Rosen RC et al. The process of care model for evaluation and treatment of erectile dysfunction. The process of care consensus panel. International Journal of Impotence Research. 1999;**11**:59-70. https://www.ncbi.nlm.nih.gov/pubmed/10356665

[56] Althof SE et al. Standard operating procedures for taking a sexual history. The Journal of Sexual Medicine. 2013;**10**:26 https://www.ncbi.nlm.nih.gov/pubmed/22970717

[57] Rosen RC et al. The international index of erectile function (IIEF): A multidimensional scale for assessment of erectile dysfunction. Urology. 1997;**49**:822 https://www.ncbi.nlm.nih.gov/pubmed/9187685

[58] World Health Organisation (ICD-10). International Statistical Classification of Diseases and Related Health Problems. Geneva: WHO; 1992

[59] McCabe MP et al. Definitions of sexual dysfunctions in women and men: A consensus statement from the fourth international consultation on sexual medicine 2015. The Journal of Sexual Medicine. 2016;**13**(2):135-143

[60] Graham CA. The DSM diagnostic criteria for female orgasmic disorder. Archives of Sexual Behavior. 2010;**39**(2):256-270

[61] Hatzichristou DG et al. Hemodynamic characterization of a functional erection: Arterial and corporeal veno-occlusive function in patients with a positive intracavernosal injection test. European Urology. 1999;**36**:60

[62] Sikka SC et al. Standardization of vascular assessment of erectile dysfunction: Standard operating procedures for duplex ultrasound. The Journal of Sexual Medicine. 2013;**10**:120 https://www.ncbi.nlm.nih.gov/pubmed/22970798

[63] Glina S et al. SOP: Corpus cavernosum assessment (cavernosography/cavernosometry). The Journal of Sexual Medicine. 2013;**10**:111 https://www.ncbi.nlm.nih.gov/pubmed/22971225

[64] Hatzichristou D et al. Recommendations for the clinical evaluation of men and women with sexual dysfunction. The Journal of Sexual Medicine. 2010;**7**:337 https://www.ncbi.nlm.nih.gov/pubmed/20092443

[65] Capogrosso P et al. One patient out of four with newly diagnosed erectile dysfunction is a young man--worrisome picture from the everyday clinical practice. The Journal of Sexual Medicine. 2013;**10**:1833 https://www.ncbi.nlm.nih.gov/pubmed/23651423

[66] Buvat J et al. Endocrine aspects of male sexual dysfunctions. The Journal of Sexual Medicine. 2010;**7**:1627 https://www.ncbi.nlm.nih.gov/pubmed/20388162

[67] Köhler TS, McVary KT. The relationship between erectile dysfunction and lower urinary tract symptoms and the role of phosphodiesterase type 5 inhibitors. European Urology. 2009;**55**:38-48

[68] Gacci M et al. Critical analysis of the relationship between sexual dysfunctions and lower urinary tract symptoms due to benign prostatic hyperplasia. European Urology. 2011;**60**:809-825

[69] Rantell A et al. How does lower urinary tract dysfunction affect sexual function in men and women? ICI-RS 2015-part 1. Neurourology and Urodynamics. 2017;**36**:949-952

[70] Giona S, Ganguly I, Muir G. Urologists' attitudes to sexual complications of LUTS/BPH treatments. World of Journal Urology. 2018;**36**:1449-1145

[71] Gacci M, Corona G, Salvi M, et al. A systematic review and meta-analysis on the use of phosphodiesterase 5 inhibitors alone or in combination with α-blockers for lower urinary tract symptoms due to benign prostatic hyperplasia. European Urology. 2012;**61**(5):994-1003

[72] van Dijk MM, de la Rosette JJ, Michel MC. E ects of alpha (1)-adrenoceptor antagonists on male sexual function. Drugs. 2006;**66**:287-301

[73] Roehrborn CG, Siami P, Barkin J, et al. The in uence of baseline parameters on changes in international prostate symp- tom score with dutasteride, tamsulosin, and combination therapy among men with symptomatic benign prostatic hyperplasia and an enlarged prostate: 2-year data from the CombAT study. European Urology. 2009;**55**:461-471

[74] Roehrborn CG, Boyle P, Nickel JC, et al. Efficacy and safety of a dual inhibitor of 5-alpha-reductase types 1 and 2 (dutasteride) in men with benign prostatic hyperplasia. Urology. 2002;**60**:434-441

[75] Roehrborn CG, Siami P, Barkin J, et al. The e ects of dutas- teride, tamsulosin and combination therapy on lower urinary tract symptoms in men with benign prostatic hyperplasia and pros- tatic enlargement: 2-year results from the CombAT study. The Journal of Urology. 2008;**179**:616-621

[76] McConnell JD, Roehrborn CG, Bautista OM, et al. The long-term e ect of doxazosin, nasteride, and combination ther- apy on the clinical progression of benign prostatic hyperplasia. The New England Journal of Medicine. 2003;**349**:2387-2398

[77] Roehrborn CG, Siami P, Barkin J, et al. The effects of combination therapy with dutasteride and tamsulosin on clinical outcomes in men with symptomatic benign prostatic hyperplasia: 4-year results from the CombAT study. European Urology. 2010;**83**:227-237;57:123-131

[78] Naslund MJ, Miner M. A review of the clinical efficacy and safety of 5alpha-reductase inhibitors for the enlarged prostate. Clinical Therapeutics. 2007;**29**(1):17-25

[79] Madersbacher S, Marberger M. Is transurethral resection of the prostate still justified? BJU International. 1999

[80] McConnell JD, Barry MJ, Bruskewitz RC. Benign prostatic hyperplasia: Diagnosis and treatment In: (AHCPR) AfHCPaR (ed), Clinical Practice Guideline Quick Reference, Guide for Clinicians. 1994;**8**:1-17

[81] Emberton M, Neal DE, Black N, et al. The effect of prostatectomy on symptom severity and quality of life. British Journal of Urology. 1996;77:233-247

[82] Horasanli K, Silay MS, Altay B, Tanriverdi O, Sarica K, Miroglu C. Photoselective potassium titanyl phosphate (KTP) laser vaporization versus transurethral resection of the prostate for prostates larger than 70 ml: A short-term prospective randomized trial. Urology. 2008;**71**:247-251

[83] Alivizatos G, Skolarikos A, Chalikopoulos D, et al. Transurethral photoselective vaporization versus transvesical open enucleation for prostatic adenomas >80 ml: 12-mo results of a randomized prospective study. European Urology. 2008;**54**:427-437

[84] Bouchier-Hayes DM, Anderson P, Van Appledorn S, Bugeja P, Costello AJ. KTP laser versus transurethral resection: Early results of a randomized trial. Journal of Endourology. 2006;**20**:580-585

[85] Naspro R, Suardi N, Salonia A, et al. Holmium laser enucleation of the prostate versus open prostatectomy for prostates >70 g: 24-month follow-up. European Urology. 2006;**50**:563-568

[86] Briganti A, Naspro R, Gallina A, et al. Impact on sexual function of holmium laser enucleation versus transurethral resection of the prostate: Results of a prospective, 2-center, randomized trial. The Journal of Urology. 2006;**175**:1817-1821

[87] Tabatabaei S, Choi B, Muir G. 2272 ejaculation-preserving

photo-selective vaporization of prostate (EP-PVP): Six years experience from a multi-Centre study. The Journal of Urology. 2011;**185**:e910-e911

[88] Kim M, Song SH, Ku JH, Kim HJ, Paick JS. Pilot study of the clinical efficacy of ejaculatory hood sparing technique for ejaculation preservation in holmium laser enucleation of the prostate. International Journal of Impotence Research. 2014;**27**:20-24

[89] Bruskewitz R, Issa MM, Roehrborn CG, et al. A prospective, randomized 1-year clinical trial comparing transurethral needle ablation to transurethral resection of the prostate for the treatment of symptomatic benign prostatic hyperplasia. The Journal of Urology. 1998;**159**:1588-1593

[90] Hill B, Belville W, Bruskewitz R, et al. Transurethral needle ablation versus transurethral resection of the prostate for the treatment of symptomatic benign prostatic hyperplasia: 5-year results of a prospective, randomized, multicenter clinical trial. The Journal of Urology. 2004;**171**:2336-2340

[91] Cimentepe E, Unsal A, Saglam R. Randomized clinical trial comparing transurethral needle ablation with transurethral resection of the prostate for the treatment of benign prostatic hyperplasia: Results at 18 months. Journal of Endourology/Endourological Society. 2003;**17**:103

[92] Woo HH, Chin PT, McNicholas TA, et al. Safety and feasibility of the prostatic urethral lift: A novel, minimally invasive treatment for lower urinary tract symptoms (LUTS) secondary to benign prostatic hyperplasia (BPH). BJU International. 2011;**108**:82-88

[93] Filippi S, Morelli A, Sandner P, et al. Characterization and functional role of androgen-dependent PDE5 activity in the bladder. Endocrinology. 2007;**148**(3):1019-1029

[94] Fibbi B, Morelli A, Vignozzi L, et al. Characterization of phosphodiesterase type 5 expression and functional activity in the human male lower urinary tract. The Journal of Sexual Medicine. 2010;**7**(1 Pt 1):59-69

[95] Morelli A, Filippi S, Comeglio P, et al. Acute vardenal administration improves bladder oxygenation in spontaneously hypertensive rats. The Journal of Sexual Medicine. 2010;**7**(1 Pt 1):107-120

[96] Morelli A, Sarchielli E, Comeglio P, et al. Phosphodiesterase type 5 expression in human and rat lower urinary tract tissues and the effect of tadalafil on prostate gland oxygenation in spontaneously hypertensive rats. The Journal of Sexual Medicine. 2011;**8**(10):2746-2760

[97] McVary KT, Roehrborn CG, Kaminetsky JC, et al. Tadalafil relieves lower urinary tract symptoms secondary to benign prostatic hyperplasia. The Journal of Urology. 2007;**177**(4):1401-1407

[98] İrer B et al. Evaluation of sexual dysfunction, lower urinary tract symptoms and quality of life in men with obstructive sleep apnea syndrome and the efficacy of continuous positive airway pressure therapy. Urology. 2018;**121**:86-92

[99] Miyazato M, Tohyama K, Touyama M, et al. Effect of continuous positive airway pressure on nocturnal urine production in patients with obstructive sleep apnea syndrome. Neurourology and Urodynamics. 2017;**36**:376-379

[100] Campos-Juanatey FF, Fernandez-Barriales M, Gonzalez M, Portillo-Martin JA. Effects of obstructive sleep apnea and its treatment over the erectile function: A systematic review. Asian Journal of Andrology. 2017;**19**:303-310